SPEECH AND LANGUAGE

SPEECH AND LANGUAGE
Detecting and Correcting
Special Needs

Joyce S. Choate/Series Consulting Editor
Northeast Louisiana University

PAULETTE J. THOMAS
University of New Orleans

FAIRY F. CARMACK
*Speech/Language Pathologist,
Monroe, Louisiana*

ALLYN AND BACON
Boston / London / Sydney / Toronto

THE ALLYN AND BACON
DETECTING AND CORRECTING SERIES
Joyce S. Choate, *Series Consulting Editor*

Editorial Production Service: Karen G. Mason
Copyeditor: Susan Freese
Cover Administrator: Linda K. Dickinson
Cover Designer: Susan Slovinsky

Library of Congress Cataloging-in-Publication Data

Thomas, Paulette J.
      Speech and language.
      (The Allyn and Bacon detecting and correcting series)
      1. Speech therapy   I. Carmack, Fairy R.   II. Title.
III. Series
RC423.T48   1989   616.85'5   89-18260

ISBN 0-205-12364-3

Printed in the United States of America

10 9 8 7 6 5 4 3 2 1   94 93 92 91 90 89

Contents

FOREWORD
ABOUT THE DETECTING AND CORRECTING SERIES

Speech and Language: Detecting and Correcting Special Needs is one of several books in an affordable series that focuses on the classroom needs of special students, both exceptional and nonexceptional, who often require adjusted methods and curricula. The purpose of this book, as well as the others in the series, is to supplement more comprehensive and theoretical treatments of major instructional issues—in this case, improving speech and language skills—with practical classroom practices.

The underlying theme of each book in the *Detecting and Correcting* series is targeted instruction to maximize students' achievement. Designed for informed teachers and teachers-in-training who are responsible for instructing special students in a variety of settings, these books emphasize the application of theory to everyday classroom concerns. While this approach may not be unique, the format in which both theme and purpose are presented is in that it enables the reader to quickly translate theory into practical classroom strategies for reaching hard-to-teach students.

Each book begins with an overview of instruction in the given subject, addressing in particular the needs of special students. The groundwork is laid here for both Detection and Correction: observing students' difficulties and then designing individualized prescriptive programs. Remaining chapters are organized into sequentially numbered units, addressing specific skill and topical needs of special students. Each unit follows a consistent two-part format. Detection is addressed first, beginning with a citation of a few significant behaviors and continuing with a discussion of factors such as descriptions and implications. The second part of each unit is Correction, which offers a number of strategies for modification according to individual students' learning needs.

This simple, consistent format makes the *Detecting and Correcting* books accessible and easy to read. Other useful features include: a) the Contents organization, designed for quick location of appropriate topics and problem skills and behaviors; b) a concise explanation of skills, special needs, and guiding principles for implementing instruction; c) a "Reflections" section ending each part, providing discussion and application activities; and d) an index of general topics and cross-references to related subjects.

Speech and language, perhaps even more so than reading (the topic of the a closely related book), empower students to learn and thus represents a major area in which special students often require special accommodations. Together, these and the other related books on basic mathematics, classroom behavior, instructional management, language arts, science and health, and social studies comprise an expanding series that simplifies teachers' tasks by offering sound and practical classroom procedures for detecting and correcting special needs.

Joyce S. Choate
Series Consulting Editor

PREFACE

Speech and Language: Detecting and Correcting Special Needs is designed to address the communication needs of exceptional and nonexceptional students. As a resource for practicing speech/language pathologists and a supplementary text in college classes, it is intended for use by teachers, prospective teachers and speech/language pathologists, and prospective speech/language pathologists who are concerned with improving the communication skills of students in both regular and special education classroom settings. The format of this book is deliberately brief and concise in order to serve as a resource from which teaching strategies and practice exercises can be easily extracted. The intent is to enable the reader to quickly translate speech and language theories into practical classroom strategies to improve the verbal and nonverbal communication skills of special students.

ASSUMPTIONS

In this text, special students include both formally identified exceptional learners and nonexceptional learners who demonstrate difficulty with speech and/or language. The basic assumptions underlying the structure and content of the book are the following:

- Language is the basis for all learning in academic settings and in the community at large.
- Normal speech and language development proceed in an orderly, somewhat predictable sequence.
- If presented appropriately, communication skills can be taught to those who exhibit incorrect, incomplete, or absent language production.
- Since students must use communication skills throughout the day, the responsibility for improving these skills resides with therapists, teachers, and parents with whom students interact daily.
- An integral part of corrective instruction encompasses opportunities for the student to apply newly acquired skills in natural settings.

These assumptions are incorporated into the Detection and Correction model for identifying the special speech and language needs of individual students and then correcting those needs by providing carefully constructed strategies for acquiring and practicing appropriate communication skills.

ORGANIZATION

The Table of Contents is designed to provide an at-a-glance guide to quickly locate the specific speech and language needs of special students. In order to avoid sex-related stereotyping, the authors have systematically alternated gender references across discussions and skills. Thus, beginning with Chapter 4, even-numbered skills use feminine pronouns and odd-numbered skills use masculine pronouns. For ease of reference and discussion, categories of speech and language needs are enumerated. Although labeled as discrete classifications, it is important to remember that rarely do these categorizations exist in a vacuum. The Table of Contents also provides a menu from which to select activities that may prove useful with speech/language-impaired youngsters.

The text is divided into five major parts. Each begins with an introductory overview and concludes with suggestions for reflecting on the content. Readers will find "Reflections" helpful for considering and extending their understandings while college instructors will find the activities particularly useful for clarification, discussion, and application as well. In each part, the final "Reflections" item refers to additional resource for further information.

Part I lays the foundation for understanding and implementing the Detection and Correction procedures suggested throughout the book. Chapter 1 briefly describes the speech process, and the language process is outlined in the second chapter. Chapter 3 addresses special communication needs of special populations. Part II is devoted to Detection and Correction strategies associated with articulation of consonants, vowels, and diphthongs. Part III contains strategies for detecting and correcting deviations in voice and includes suggestions to modify voice pitch, intensity, and quality. Part IV is devoted to identifying and remediating disorders of fluency, including stuttering and cluttering. Part V presents strategies for detecting and correcting the verbal communication disorders of semantics, morphology, syntax, word finding, and special language problems. Part V also includes suggestions for identifying and remediating disorders of nonverbal communication. An Appendix lists symbols of the International Phonetic Alphabet and a key word associated with each.

FEATURES

These strategies for detecting and correcting communication disorders are founded in theory and translated into practice. The strategies reflect the successful practice of the authors and their associates. The exercises contain ordinary words and phrases as well as those that are semantically interesting. The activities are geared to a wide age and intellectual functioning range. The user is encouraged to modify procedures according to the student's age, needs, and interests. Most of the strategies can be implemented in both regular and special education settings with individuals and both small and large groups of students. Because the strategies must be adapted to fit individual students and teachers/pathologists only the most salient features are described. To keep the text clear, succinct, and practical, speech and language theory is built into the strategies.

As an instantly useful study and reference aid, a consistent format is used throughout. Every chapter includes a diagnostic section entitled Detection and a prescriptive teaching section entitled Correction. In Chapters 4 through 16, the discussion of the Detection and Correction of speech and language needs is presented on two facing pages. Each treatment begins with a list of a few observable behaviors that may signal a special need for instruction in the particular skill. Next is a description of the skill and of the problems students often exhibit. The possible causes for the speech or language impairment and the implications for continued errors are mentioned. Several strategies are suggested for correcting each problem. Many of these corrective strategies are also appropriate for most students, but it is the special students who must have the special instruction in order to improve communication skills.

ACKNOWLEDGMENTS

These strategies reflect the authors' accumulated experience with numerous speech/language students; we acknowledge each of those students and the invaluable lessons they have taught us. We appreciate the expertise of Kaye Eichler, who contributed the majority of the content of the chapter on fluency, and Jorenda R. Stone, for technical assistance in the microcomputer lab.

For painstakingly reviewing the manuscript and providing guidance we are grateful to our field reviewers: Anthony Baschir (Children's Hospital and Boston College); Leah Lorendo (Northeastern University); and Phyllis Lubar (Needham Public Schools, Massachusetts).

We gratefully acknowledge the untiring effort of Joyce Choate, Series Consulting Editor, to bring this project to fruition. A special thank you is due our editorial team at Allyn and Bacon: Mylan Jaixen, Ray Short, and Karen Mason. We express appreciation to our friends and colleagues who supported our endeavor and seemed to understand our preoccupation with "the book." And to our families, who have not shown any permanent effects of benign neglect, we send our love and gratitude.

PART I

SPECIAL SPEECH AND
LANGUAGE NEEDS

Humans are social creatures who must interact with other humans in order to survive. Indeed, as Harlow discovered decades ago in his experiments with primates, infant monkeys who were exposed to noncommunicative, wire monkeys developed aberrant behaviors. In human infants, a phenomenon known as *marasmus* was detected and described early in this century. Human infants who were institutionalized and experienced a minimal amount of human contact often died or failed to thrive because of lack of human attention. Although marasmus is an extreme form of isolation, it is nonetheless a poignant illustration of the need for human contact. This need is generally satisfied through verbal and nonverbal communication. Verbal communication may take the form of speaking, reading, or writing; nonverbal communication may be expressed through prosody, gestures, facial expression, body posture, and proxemics. There must be a mutually agreed upon language system in order for communication to occur. Without a means of communication, an individual becomes a social isolate and is likely to be disturbed.

Speech is the means by which we transmit thoughts that are generate
our system of language. Speech is disordered when it calls unfavorable atte
to the speaker, hinders the communication process, or causes maladjustment
in the speaker. The speaker whose speech is disordered may exhibit deficiencies in articulation, voice, and/or fluency. Articulation is disordered when
substitutions, distortions, omissions, and/or additions of speech sounds are of
such magnitude that the speaker cannot be fully understood or the communication process is impaired. Voice is considered disordered when pitch, loudness,
and/or quality deviate to such an extent as to be inappropriate to sex, age, or
cultural expectations. Fluency disorders occur when the natural rhythm and flow
of speech is interrupted by repetitions, prolongations, and/or hesitations.

With speech as the vehicle for communication, language is the raw material
that serves as the impetus to communicate and provides the building blocks for
our communication system. Components of verbal language include semantics
(word meanings), morphology (a rule system that governs changes that modify
meaning at the word level), syntax (the rules that govern the ordering of words
in sentences), and vocabulary (the bank from which words are selected).
Nonverbal language extends meaning and serves to confirm, deny, or emphasize oral language. Nonverbal communication includes prosody, kinesics, and
proxemics.

Special-needs students may exhibit disordered communicative behaviors
that are associated with their particular handicapping conditions. Cerebral-
palsied, hearing-impaired, learning-disabled, cleft palate, mentally retarded,
behavior-disordered, visually impaired, and physically handicapped individuals
are likely to display types of communication disorders that will require specially
designed intervention. There are, additionally, age-related disorders that may
necessitate therapeutic measures.

The communication needs of the exceptional student are not defined by the
category of handicapping condition. Rather, each special-needs student exhibits communication behaviors unique to himself or herself. It is the perceptive
teacher or therapist who is able to exactly determine the particular communication need of the individual student and select appropriate strategies for improvement. Since communication is the window to the self, it is vitally important that
each special-needs student participate in exercises designed to improve and
enhance his or her communication ability.

Chapters 1, 2, and 3 present in some detail descriptive, developmental, and
therapeutic techniques of numerous communication disorders. These chapters
provide more elaborate descriptions of developmental aspects of speech and
language than can be found in the skill treatments. Selected references are listed
in the Reflections section for those readers who wish an even more complete
treatise on selected topics.

CHAPTER 1

THE SPEECH PROCESS

The terms *communication, language,* and *speech* often are erroneously used synonymously or interchangeably. The distinctions among these three terms are presented in this book. Communication and language descriptions are detailed in Chapter 2. The description and development of speech are addressed in this chapter.

SPEECH PRODUCTION

Speech is the means by which oral communication takes place. The act of speaking requires precise neuromuscular coordination of the organs of speech and the messages sent and received by the brain. Speech is a voluntary act that occurs as a result of the activation of respiration, phonation, and articulation. The structures (anatomy) of the speech mechanism will be described briefly, and then the process (physiology) of speech production will be described briefly.

The lower respiratory tract encompasses the diaphragm, lungs, and trachea. The upper respiratory tract includes the larynx, pharynx, and oral and nasal cavities. The vocal tract includes the throat (pharynx), mouth (oral cavity), and nasal cavities. The articulators are the tongue, soft and hard palates, teeth, lips, and jaw.

The most simple description of the process of speech is that it follows the sequence of respiration, phonation, resonation, and articulation. Air is exhaled from the lungs to the trachea. The passage of exhaled air is stopped momentarily by the coming together of the vocal folds (adduction), which allows for an increase in the air pressure of the exhaled air. The resistance of the vocal folds is overcome and a puff of air is released. The air vibrates the vocal cords and produces sound. The sound is resonated in the oral cavity and shaped into speech sounds by the articulators.

Although described here in simple terms, speech is an extremely complex process that can be disrupted by any number of factors, including neuromuscular disorders (cerebral palsy), obstructive airway conditions (asthma), lung tissue disorders (emphysema), structural anomalies (cleft palate), laryngeal pathologies (vocal nodules), and paralysis of any of the structures necessary for speech.

Articulation Development

The smallest unit of speech is the phoneme, or speech sound. Each language has its own set of phonemes and combinations of phonemes that are characteristic of that language. Phonemes are combined in specific ways to form words. In the English language, phonological rules govern the ways in which phonemes can be combined. For example, [ŋ] never appears at the beginning of a word, [h] and [j] never appear at the end of a word, and [t] can appear almost anywhere in a word. Similarly, *dring* is not a recognized word in the English language, but *drink* is. *Brush* and *brash* are recognized, but *brosh* and *brish* are not.

In the English language, phonemes are classified as vowels or consonants. Vowels are produced with a relatively open vocal tract that allows for a continuous, unrestricted airflow. Consonants, on the other hand, are produced by creating constrictions in various places and degrees in the vocal tract. Phonemes can be described as voiced or voiceless. Voiced phonemes are produced by the vibration of the vocal folds. The vocal folds do not vibrate when voiceless phonemes are produced. All vowels in the English language are voiced. Consonants may be voiced or voiceless. The strategies for DETECTION and CORRECTION in Chapter 4 indicate which phonemes are voiced and which are voiceless.

The traditional phonemic classification system has been selected for use in this book. This classification system is based on the place of articulation (and, for consonants, the manner of articulation) and voicing. The place of articulation describes the position where the maximum constriction occurs and includes the following descriptors:

consonants	vowels
bilabial	front
glottal	back
labiodental	central
lingua-alveolar	high
linguadental	mid
linguapalatal	low
linguavelar	

Descriptions and examples of these descriptors are found in Chapter 4.

The manner of articulation generally describes the degree of constriction of the vocal tract and the type of release of air. The descriptors associated with the manner of articulation include plosive, fricative, nasal, affricate, liquid, and glide. A more complete discussion of manner of articulation is presented in Chapter 4. Voicing is indicated for each consonant included in Chapter 4, Skills 1 through 16.

Speech Development

Just as there are developmental milestones in physical development, there are also developmental milestones in the development of speech as a communication device. The newborn makes nondifferentiated cries and vegetative sounds. The noncrying sounds uttered include normal phonation but incomplete resonance in the oral cavity. Sounds tend to be quite nasal because much air is emitted through the nasal cavity.

The infant enters the cooing stage around 2 months of age. She is able to produce back consonants and mid and back vowel sounds, but resonation is still incomplete. Velopharyngeal closure (the separating of the oral from the nasal cavity by action of the soft palate and the pharyngeal walls) is approximated so that the airstream is directed into the oral cavity rather than into the nasal cavity.

The baby usually begins babbling around age 4 months. She gains greater control of her tongue and vocalizes for prolonged periods of time. She begins to experiment with sound production, often producing sounds that do not appear in her native language. Labials (sounds that require bringing the lips together) emerge as preferred sounds ("ma-ma") by 6 months. Between 6 and 10 months, the infant's babbling becomes reduplicated strings of consonant-vowel syllables ("ba-ba-ba"). Labial and alveolar plosives are emerging as well as nasals. (Plosives are sounds that are made by obstructing the airstream and then releasing it quickly, resulting in a little explosion; alveolar describes the place of articulation, the gum ridge; nasals are sounds formed when the airstream exits via the nasal cavity rather than the oral cavity.) During the 11- to 14-month period, speech is characterized by babbling in which adjacent syllables are not identical. The child frequently strings together syllables with intonational patterns that are unintelligible (jargon) but may imitate adult statements or questions. First words emerge about this time. Development at this stage is dependent upon gaining conscious control of the articulators and learning the associations between objects and their labels.

ACQUISITION OF SPEECH SOUNDS

Several researchers have attempted to discover the order of acquisition of speech sounds. To date, there is not a universally accepted norm within which phonemes are acquired. There are, however, several general conclusions that may be drawn and a range of development within which phoneme production occurs.

1. As a group, vowels are acquired before consonants and are usually acquired by age 3.
2. The manner of articulation of consonants follows a certain order of acquisition:

    nasals—sounds produced when the soft palate is lowered to allow the airstream to exit via the nasal cavity

    glides—sounds produced while gliding from one vowel position to another

    plosives—sounds produced when the airstream is obstructed and then released quickly

    liquids—consonant sounds that have the vowel-like quality of minor air turbulence in the oral cavity

    fricatives—sounds produced by constricting the air passage so that the air must exit through a narrow channel

    affricates—sounds produced by the combination of a fricative following a plosive

3. The place of articulation of consonants follows a certain order of acquisition:

(?) *h*   *glottals*—restriction occurs at the glottis②

m pb ⦿⦿*bi* *labials*—the lips are brought together ②

ŋ kg   *velars*—constriction occurs when the back of the tongue contacts the soft palate (velum)

n l sz t d *alveolars*—the place of constriction is the front of the tongue to the gum (alveolar) ridge

dentals—the constriction occurs when the lower lip is

fv   brought to the upper teeth (labiodental) or when the

⦿⦿ *θ ʒ* tongue tip is brought to the upper teeth (linguadental)—*interdentals*

ʃʒ tʃ dʒ rj *palatals*—the place of constriction is the tongue on the hard palate

4. Sounds are acquired first in the initial position in words.

5. Consonant clusters and blends are not acquired until age 7 or 8, but some clusters are noted at age 4.

6. Individual differences may account for normal variation of phoneme acquisition. (Shames & Wiig, 1987)

For more than three decades, researchers have investigated the age at which consonant sounds are normally acquired. One researcher (Sandler, 1972) analyzed the data of several investigators and developed an age range of speech sound acquisition of consonants. The lower age represents the age at which 50% of children pronounced the tested consonant sound correctly in two positions in words. The upper age indicates the age at which 90% of the children tested produced the target sound in all three positions in words. In Chapter 4, under DETECTION, the behavior that is described is, in all cases, attached to an age. That age is presented here as the age at which 90% of the youngsters pronounce the sound in all three word positions. It follows then that only about 10% of the population will either be delayed in acquisition of consonants or will not spontaneously pronounce the target sound without intervention.

phoneme	50%; 2/3 word positions	90%; 3/3 word positions
[p]	<2	3
[m]	<2	3
[h]	<2	3
[n]	<2	3
[w]	<2	3
[b]	<2	4
[k]	2	4
[g]	2	4
[d]	2	4
[t]	2	6
[n]	2	6
[f]	2 1/2	4

phoneme	50%; 2/3 word positions	90%; 3/3 word positions
[j]	2 1/2	4
[r]	3	6
[l]	3	6
[s]	3	8
[tʃ]	3 1/2	7
[ʃ]	3 1/2	7
[z]	3 1/2	8
[dʒ]	4	7
[v]	4	8
[θ]	4 1/2	7
[ð]	5	8
[ʒ]	6	8 1/2

This developmental information provides broad guidelines for consonant acquisition. Individual children may vary considerably within the guidelines. Consideration should always be given to the child's intelligibility before seeking corrective measures. Compare the misarticulated sounds with the age ranges presented here to determine the approximate range of normal. Professional help should definitely be sought if the student does not correctly pronounce the phonemes at the same relative age as 90% of his peers. Remember that children may vary greatly in many aspects of physical, intellectual, and social development. The presence of handicapping conditions may inhibit or delay the acquisition of speech sounds.

Detection of Articulation Errors

There are four types of articulation errors: substitution, distortion, omission, and addition. Substitution errors occur when the intended phoneme is replaced by another phoneme (e.g., *wed* instead of *red*). An articulation error that is classified as a distortion occurs when the phoneme sounds different but not different enough to be recognized as another phoneme (e.g., lateral lisp). A phoneme that is absent and that should be pronounced is described as an omission (e.g., *hambur_er*). An infrequent articulation error, where superfluous sounds are inserted, is termed an addition error (*hippomapotamus*).

Typically, these articulation errors occur with consonants, not vowels. The most usual vowel problem is distortion. When vowels are misarticulated, it is usually the result of some type of organic disorder such as cerebral palsy or paralysis of the articulators, hearing impairment, severe mental retardation, or primary language other than English.

In this book, the DETECTION section of Chapter 4 details the age at which 90% of children have mastered the target sound, voicing, manner of articulation, and place of articulation. This section includes a description of the sounds, possible reasons the misarticulation occurs, and implications for failure to produce the sounds correctly.

Correction of Articulation Errors

The CORRECTION sections follow the traditional sequence of speech therapy. The first activity in each skill is auditory discrimination. The second activity presented is production in isolation. This section includes explicit directions for teaching the student how to produce the target sound. Suggestions are detailed for guiding the student to practice production in nonsense syllables/words and production in phrases/sentences. Creative and interesting generalization activities are included to be performed in three settings: in class, at home, and in the community. Sample words, phrases, and sentences are provided for all articulation skills. The vowel and diphthong chapter (5) describes proper placement of the articulators and offers sample words for practice.

ASPECTS OF VOICE

The pitch, loudness, and quality of the voice play an important role in the communication process. The content and organization of speech are enhanced or discounted oftentimes by the way the speaker sounds. Since many professions rely heavily on being able to convey feelings and thoughts effectively, adults are probably highly motivated to seek help for voice disorders. Similarly, many parents are quite interested in exploring assistance for their children who have voice problems so as not to limit their professional options.

Detection of Voice Disorders

Voice is considered to be disordered when it consistently deviates in pitch, loudness, or quality from that which is expected for age, sex, and culture. Deviations in pitch occur when the vibratory frequency of the voice is either too high, too low, or without adequate variation. Loudness disorders are noted when the volume of speech is either too loud or too soft; either may indicate the presence of a sensorineural or conductive hearing loss. The most frequently exhibited voice disorder is deviation in voice quality. Vocal quality that is hoarse, nasal, or breathy presents a challenge to the practitioner because of the complex nature of the disorder.

Voice disorders may stem from functional or organic causes or a combination of the two. Functional causes may include disturbances of personality that are reflected in the voice, poor speech models for imitation so that the child learns poor vocal habits through the normal process of learning, and poor vocalization habits. Organic causes may include anomalies in the structure of the vocal mechanism, poor physical health, laryngeal pathologies, and/or hearing impairments that would affect the individual's ability to monitor his voice during speech. Since phonation occurs within the larynx, the action of the vocal folds is not easily observed either directly or indirectly without sophisticated instruments. And because the course of treatment or therapy is different depending on the etiology of the voice disorder, it is *always* necessary to obtain a diagnosis from a physician (preferably an otolaryngologist) before any treatment or therapy is initiated. Failure to obtain medical clearance is not only a breach of ethics for the speech pathologist but a potentially dangerous situation for the client, since the diagnosis should guide the course of therapy.

Correction of Voice Disorders

Therapies may include instruction in listening skills, explanation of the process of speech (including anatomy and physiology), physical hygiene, posture and movement, regulation of respiration, relaxation, voice training, and examining and changing environmental influences. For those individuals who are not able to use the larynx for phonation due to surgical removal or injury, there are therapies that teach the individual to articulate air that is resonated either by a belch or by an artificial device.

ASPECTS OF FLUENCY

Dysfluent speech is probably the most unsettling type of speech disorder for the speaker and the listener and presents perhaps the greatest challenge for the therapist. Fluency disorders include stuttering and cluttering. Next to articulation disorders, stuttering is the most common type of speech disorder. Rare is the teacher who has taught for at least a year and not come into contact with a student who stutters. In the total population, there are four to eight times more males who stutter than females. Stuttering usually has its onset before adolescence. Those who stutter face limited vocational choices, since many professions require fluent speech for success.

Detection of Dysfluent Speech

Stuttered speech may be characterized by repetitions, prolongations, hesitations, interjections, and stuttering blocks that interrupt the smooth flow of speech. Cluttering may be described as rapid, indistinct, and arhythmic speech that may also contain repetitions. The clutterer may abruptly terminate speech sounds, omit sounds and words, and/or repeat sounds and words, all at a very rapid pace. Picture a room that is in disarray—newspapers strewn about, drinking glasses on the end table, three pairs of tennis shoes in varying sizes on the floor. Now put that scene into motion with the objects moving in rapid, staccato bursts. If that visual image could be translated to speech, you would have a very good idea of cluttered speech.

Numerous theories exist regarding the cause of dysfluent speech. No one universally accepted theory explains why all dysfluent speakers become dysfluent speakers. Many therapies have been developed from these causation theories. The strategies in this book adopt those therapies that have been shown to be effective in reducing fluency disorders.

Correction of Dysfluent Speech

In considering fluency disorders, it is important to remember that everyone is normally dysfluent occasionally. No one is dysfluent all the time. Another rule of thumb is that most children between the ages of 3 and 5 exhibit dysfluencies that should be considered normal. It is also interesting to note that stutterers usually do not stutter when reciting a well-known poem or singing a song.

The best course of preventive action is to focus on the message being sent and ignore the dysfluencies. Do not call attention to the dysfluencies or, according to behaviorists, you will assist that child in becoming a stutterer. The preferable response to dysfluent speech is to continue to listen and maintain eye contact; do not finish the speaker's thoughts for him, and do not instruct him to "spit it out!" Numerous effective strategies for decreasing dysfluencies are contained in Chapters 9 and 10. Some of the skills in these chapters focus on changing and creating response patterns and identifying possible stress situations. All the skills are geared toward the goal of reducing dysfluencies, thereby improving the communicative process.

SUMMARY

This chapter contains information explaining the structures of the speech mechanism and the process by which speech physically occurs. The traditional phonemic classification system was used to describe production of consonants and vowels. Acquisition of speech sounds was presented according to manner of articulation, place of articulation, and chronological age at which most youngsters have acquired use of specific phonemes. The four types of articulation errors were presented and examples of each given. The reader was referred to specific skills for specific DETECTION and CORRECTION activities.

This chapter also discussed the less frequently occurring speech disorders of voice and fluency. Pitch, loudness, and quality were introduced as the aspects of voice that may be disordered. The reader was cautioned to *always* seek a medical opinion before beginning any type of voice therapy or correction. The fluency disorders, stuttering and cluttering, were briefly described. Some preventive actions were given to assist in maintaining fluency.

THE LANGUAGE PROCESS

COMMUNICATION

Communication is the process of transmission and reception of (or representing and receiving of) information. This definition implies that: 1) Communication is active, not passive, and is a process, not a product; and 2) Communication is an interaction that involves a sender (or speaker) and a receiver (or listener). Communication may be interindividual or intraindividual.

Interindividual Communication

Interindividual communication occurs between two or more people and is not restricted to live dialogue. Examples of interindividual communication include:

Conversation between two individuals. This type of interindividual communication sees the participants in alternating roles of transmitter and receiver. Speaker 1 initiates the conversation and is the transmitter while speaker 2 is the listener or receiver. When speaker 2 responds, he becomes the transmitter and speaker 1 the receiver. If speaker 1 elects to respond, she again becomes the transmitter and speaker 2 the receiver, and so forth.

Television, radio, or film transmission. These broadcasts are also considered to be interindividual communication. They are, however, one-way communications. There is still a transmitter (the actor, news broadcaster, commentator) and a receiver (the audience, listener), but the participants do not change roles.

Written communication. Written communication may take the form of letter writing between correspondents or reading a novel or article. With letter writing, the correspondents take the alternating roles of transmitter, receiver, transmitter, receiver, and so on. In the act of reading, the reader is the receiver and the author is the transmitter. The reader may decide to respond to the author, perhaps writing a letter to the editor in response to a newspaper article, and then becomes the transmitter. The author of the newspaper article may or may not become the receiver.

Intraindividual Communication

Intraindividual communication occurs within one person, who is both transmitter and receiver. The purposes of intraindividual communication include language to plan, rehearse, self-regulate, and mediate. Examples of intraindividual communication include the frequent messages that we send to ourselves on a daily basis, such as internal debate over a decision.

1) "Should I run the yellow caution light? Yeah, go ahead, nobody is looking." (or "No, weather conditions are too unsafe; better not risk it.").

2) "Do I want the ice cream or the frozen yogurt? Oh, take the yogurt—it's less fattening and lower in cholesterol."

3) "Is it time to study now? Yes, I'll study now and talk on the telephone later."

Levels of Communication

Communication occurs at different levels. The three levels that will be discussed here are technical, semantic, and effective.

Technical. This level refers to how precisely symbols can be exchanged. Compare the technical quality in the following pairs of exchanges:

1) Go a couple of blocks; then turn right *versus*
   Head north on St. Charles Avenue and turn right at Canal Street.

2) Add the numbers and subtract from 100 *versus*
   Add all the numbers; subtract the sum from 100.

3) If I play this tennis match well, I can win *versus*
   I must serve well, stay in position, move my feet, come to the net on all short balls, and keep my concentration in order to beat my opponent in this tennis match.

Semantic. This level of communication refers to how precisely the symbols reflect the intended meaning. Consider the following examples:

1) *Teacher to class:* "Pay attention." The teacher's communication means that she expects all students to look at her and listen to her without talking, writing, or reading.

2) *Husband to wife:* "Please bring me a cold glass of water." The husband anticipates that his spouse will hand him water that is of low temperature served in a glass container.

3) *Candidate to electorate:* "If elected, I will not raise taxes." The political candidate expects the voters to believe that public services will be maintained and that additional revenue will come from some source other than taxation.

Effective. This level of communication refers to how precisely the receiver's response reflects the sender's intent. Illustrations may be made using the three previous examples:

1) If all students' eyes are fixated on the teacher and none of them is talking, writing, or reading, the teacher realizes that all students have understood the intent of her message (and have elected to comply with her command).

2) If the wife hands the husband a glass of water poured from the container in the refrigerator or with ice cubes in it (rather than placing a glass in the freezer to get cold), the husband observes that his communication is effective.

3) If the candidate who ran on a platform of maintaining or reducing levels of taxation is elected, the officeholder-elect understands that the voters have concluded that taxes are high enough already.

VERBAL COMMUNICATION

Verbal communication may be oral or written and involves the ability to encode and decode. *Encoding* is the process of formulating thoughts into orderly sequenced words (i.e., syntax; also see Chapter 1) in order to transmit a message. The special needs child who is language disordered may very well transmit messages in which thoughts are not arranged in the expected sequence. The necessary words may be present, but the unusual sequencing of the words will cause a breakdown in communication. Compare these two utterances: "Brad studying is for a test" versus "Brad is studying for a test."

A more innocuous example might be the native French speaker who is practicing his newly learned English. In the French language, adjectives follow nouns, whereas in the English language, the adjective usually precedes the noun. The Frenchman might say "a dress red" instead of "a red dress." Continued practice will likely result in the Frenchman's learning the more appropriate sequencing.

Decoding is the process of understanding the transmitted message and is synonymous with comprehension. The special-needs child who does not understand vocabulary and/or idiomatic expressions is at a particular disadvantage in academic and social settings. Chapters 11 through 15 present numerous strategies for assisting the special-needs learner in improving decoding and encoding abilities.

You may find it difficult to grasp the idea that some students do not understand idioms and/or vocabulary that is age appropriate. This idea may be demonstrated through the following scenario. You are watching the Monday night football game, but you do not really know very much about the rules of professional football. During one play, an official drops a yellow penalty flag. The official signals what type of penalty by holding his right fist in front of his face (palm facing his face) and lowering it a few inches. Since you are not familiar with the game, you do not know what infraction is being signaled. But help is at hand. The television commentator explains, "That was a five-yard facemask." Now you know exactly what the penalty is. Right? Well, you would if you knew the rules and vocabulary associated with professional football. Remove that visual image of a facemask that protrudes for five yards. You see, it is an infraction of the rules for one player to grab the protective facemask of another. If the infraction is deliberate or vicious, a fifteen-yard penalty is assessed against the team of the offending player. If, however, the infraction is either "accidental" or not very serious, a five-yard penalty against the team of the offending player is assessed. The observer, then, who is familiar with the rules of professional football is, therefore, easily able to decode "That was a five-yard facemask." Imagine the difficulty a special-needs child experiences when the school day is filled with words and phrases he is unable to comprehend.

In order for verbal communication to occur, the encoder and the decoder must share a similar system for representing concepts. This mutually agreed upon system or code uses arbitrary but conventional symbols whose use is governed by mutually accepted rules for combination of those symbols. This shared system is called *language.* If I said to you, "Ich habe zwei Karten für morgen nachmittag. Wollen Sie mitkommen?", you would not understand me unless you comprehend the German language. Both encoder and decoder must share the same system in order to communicate effectively.

Detection of Verbal Language Disorders

Early detection of language disorders is important to early correction of those disorders. Language is the basis of much of the learning necessary for academic success. Indeed, the student who does not understand language will experience extreme difficulty learning to read. Many reading specialists acknowledge the association between what is presented in print on the page and what is already in the speaking vocabulary of youngsters. Many teachers use the technique of writing down the student's spoken language and creating the written-spoken association as the preferred method of teaching beginning reading.

Chapters 11 through 15 describe the detection of disordered language in terms of observable behaviors. For example, the terminology used is "does not understand idioms and figurative language, single interpretation of multiple-meaning words." These behavioral descriptions are used to assist teachers, college students, and therapists to deal with problem behaviors rather than diagnostic classifications (e.g., language disordered). This type of presentation should also assist teachers and therapists in working with those who have not been classified as exceptional.

The following pages present a simple discussion of the development of understanding (receptive) and using (expressive) language. It is a generally accepted axiom that it is difficult to know what abnormal or deviant behavior is unless one is familiar with normal or typical behavior. The guidelines presented may be used as informal assessment devices if desired.

Developmental Aspects of Language Acquisition

Most of us know that we have to learn to walk before we can run. In much the same way, a youngster must understand language before she can use it. However, the process of understanding language does not have to be complete before a child uses language. Other terms that are used to describe understanding and using language that are familiar to speech-language pathologists are *receptive* and *expressive* language.

Understanding Language (Receptive Language)

There are some generally accepted milestones in the development of understanding language. The following set of questions present observable behaviors that an adult familiar with the child should be able to answer in the affirmative at the expected age. Read over the questions before doing the activity with the child. The activities require certain props to be present. If the child does not perform the actions at or near the expected age, the adult should be prepared to seek professional assistance from a speech pathologist.

By the age of	does the child . . . ?
10 months	understand name and respond?
10 months	understand "no"?
11 months	give up an object on command?
16 months	obey simple commands?
	"Give me the pencil."
	"Put the keys on the table."
	"Hand me the ball."
17 months	follow directions?
	"Put on your coat."
	"Put on your hat."
18 months	recognize and point to body parts on a doll?
	"Point to your dolly's mouth." (hands, eyes, etc.)
18 months	point out animals in pictures?
	"Where is the dog?" (cow, horse, etc.)
21 months	respond to three commands?
	"Put on your hat, pick up the book, and go to the front door."
24 months	respond to four commands?
	"Put on your hat, get your lunch box, pick up your book, and go to the front door."
27 months	understand prepositions?
	"Put this block on the table."
	"Put the ball under the chair."
	"Put the book behind me."
	"Put the cup in front of me on the floor."
36 months	respond to information about functions associated with pictured objects?
	"Point to the one that is up in the sky."
	"Point to the one that is good to eat."
	"Point to the one that is good to wear."
45 months	respond to comparative information about objects?
	"Point to the one that can swim the fastest."
	"Point to the one that is heaviest to lift."
	"Point to the one that you eat most often."

Using Language (Expressive Language)

There are also general milestones or guidelines that have been observed in children's development of language usage. Read over the checklist before attempting the exercises. Some of the activities require concrete objects or pictures. When using the checklist, keep in mind that there is a wide range of normal; moreover, some children will exhibit the described behaviors earlier than the ages listed and some will exhibit the behaviors later. If the parent, pediatrician, or teacher is concerned about the child's use of language, the best course of action is to seek professional help from a licensed speech-language pathologist.

By the age of	does the child . . . ?
12 months	imitate sounds?
12 months	combine two or more syllables?
12 months	attempt "da-da" and "ma-ma"?
18 months	have a 10- to 50-word vocabulary?
20 months	name familiar objects when shown? block, watch, keys, cup, doll, spoon
18-21 months	use two-word combinations? "Here ball," "Daddy go," "More milk"
21 months	ask for food, to go to the toilet, or drink?
21 months	use repetition of adult speech?
22 months	name familiar objects in pictures? house, dog, bird, tree, flower
24 months	use an average sentence length of two words?
24 months	frequently use three-word sentences?
24 months	refer to himself by name?
24 months	use pronouns, even though not always correctly?
24 months	beginning to use -*ing* ending?
25 months	frequently use four-word sentences?
30 months	give her full name?
30 months	refer to himself by pronoun?
30 months	give the use of familiar objects? spoon, cup, penny, keys, comb, toothbrush
30 months	use the word *is*?
30 months	use an average sentence length of over three words?
31 months	respond correctly to cause-effect questions? "What should you do when you are sleepy?" "What should you do when you are hungry?" "What should you do when you are cold?"
33 months	repeat a sentence of six syllables? "I can put on my coat." "John has a little dog."
36 months	use some plurals?
37 months	use indirect requests? "Can I get the doll?"
37 months	use an average sentence length of over four words?
40 months	use an average sentence length of 4 1/2 words?

The development of language generally proceeds from concrete to abstract and general to specific. For example, the student who is asked to talk about freedom might give a concrete or general response of "in the Pledge of Allegiance" or a more abstract or specific response of "quality of a democracy." Another example might be the response to how a cat and a mouse are similar. The concrete, general response might be that they both have four legs, a tail, and ears. The more abstract, specific response would be that they are both animals.

Correction of Verbal Language Disorders

The CORRECTION activities presented for each skill are carefully crafted to produce the desired result. The activities can be easily adapted for classrooms and single students. The exercises are written to reflect actual behaviors expected of students in school. Most students, not just the target pupil, will benefit from these skill activities.

NONVERBAL COMMUNICATION

Communication may be nonverbal or verbal. Nonverbal communication occurs in three basic categories: prosody, kinesics, and proxemics. (Some consider prosody to be a part of verbal communication.) Chapter 16 presents DETECTION and CORRECTION strategies for each of these categories.

Detection of Nonverbal Communication Disorders

Prosody
Prosodic features are variables of voice and voice use, such as pitch, duration, loudness, and rhythm. Prosodic features carry meaning and may serve to confirm or contradict the spoken message. For example, "Oh" spoken briskly with high nonvarying pitch indicates surprise. "Oh" articulated slowly, beginning with low pitch and ending with a higher pitch, indicates disbelief. And "Oh" said very slowly and of longer duration, beginning in a high pitch and ending in a lower pitch, indicates that the speaker has experienced a revelation.

Kinesics
Kinesics are visual signals sent with the body movements of gesture, facial expression, and posture. Kinesics are arbitrary movements interpreted on the basis of convention. Certain kinesics may be culture specific. For example, two unrelated American males greeting each other with kisses on both cheeks, imparts a very different message than two unrelated Italian men doing the same thing. Kinesics serve to confirm or deny the verbal

message. The employee who insists that he is open to new ideas but speaks the words while seated with legs crossed, body angled away from the boss, and arms folded tightly across the chest belies the verbal communication. In this instance, the nonverbal message denies or does not confirm the verbal message. The gentleman who is introduced to a seated lady confirms his pleasure in meeting her if he seats himself so that their eyes are on approximately the same level. Had the gentleman remained standing, he would have given an air of dominance because the lady, in order to maintain eye contact, would have been forced to assume the dominated position of head tilted backward.

The importance of kinesics in sending and receiving messages cannot be underestimated. Who of us can forget the relief we felt when greeted with open arms after having committed some childhood transgression. How different were our feelings when confronted with hands on hips and a look of disapproval? The special-needs student who does not understand or use kinesics appropriately is at a decided disadvantage, both within and outside of academic settings.

Proxemics

Proxemics describes the distance in interpersonal communication. Like kinesics, proxemics may also be culture specific. Communication that occurs at a distance of 0 to 18 inches is considered in American culture to be intimate. I like to recount the story of the behavioral research psychologist who was amusing his friends during intermission at the opera by telling about his current project: observing and recording the reactions of adult males when a male graduate student unknown to them entered their intimate distance range. The psychologist and his companions were laughing uproariously at the described reactions of the subjects. Unbeknownst to the psychologist the man whose seat was next to the psychologist's overheard the conversation. When they returned to their seats following intermission, the man cradled his chin in his hand while resting his elbow on the armrest. After a few minutes, he lifted his head from his hand, and slowly and casually let his hand drop into the psychologist's lap. I guess you can imagine the psychologist's reaction!

This anecdote illustrates American males' need to protect their intimate distance from invasion by strangers. Public distance in American culture, on the other hand, is considered to be over 12 feet. A lecturer is usually removed at least that distance from her audience. A teacher, however, purposefully closes the distance between himself and his students. But that is the nature of the two types of interactions. The lecturer's job is to present information, not necessarily to confirm that it has been learned. The teacher, however, wants to be invited into his students' intimate space so that he may function effectively.

Correction of Nonverbal Communication Disorders

The CORRECTION activities of each skill address instruction in understanding as well as using nonverbal language. Most of us learn the meanings of intonation patterns, gestures, facial expressions, postures, and appropriate distances incidentally. Many also learn the appropriate use of intonational patterns, gestures, facial expressions, postures, and appropriate distances incidentally, in the course of learning to communicate effectively. For those who have not learned these skills and/or for those who may be members of other cultures and wish to participate more fully in American culture, the skills presented should alleviate some difficulties with nonverbal communication. The skills may also prove useful for students studying acting, assisting them to convey messages nonverbally.

LANGUAGE DIFFERENCES

This section is presented to caution the reader about the distinction between *language disorders* and *language differences*. The student who exhibits language differences does not necessarily require intervention and remediation. The language-disordered student, however, does require intervention and remediation in order to experience academic success.

Language is disordered when it interferes with communication, calls unfavorable attention to itself, or causes its user to be maladjusted. A language disorder is determined within the context of a speech community. Although in the United States the common national language is English, there are a variety of speech communities. Variations of the national language are termed *dialects*. It is important to note that a dialect is not inferior, merely different. It is also true, however, that politically, socially, economically, and educationally powerful people tend to speak a standard dialect. In other words, if you want to be king, you must speak the king's English.

Seven major factors typically influence language behavior: race and ethnicity; social class, education, and occupation; region; gender; situation or context; peer group association or identification; and first language culture. Racial and ethnic influences on language are related to the cultural attitudes and values associated with group membership. Language behavior tends to reflect social class, education, and occupation. It has been generally noted that lower-class groups use a more restricted linguistic code and middle- and upper-class groups use a more elaborate linguistic code with universal meanings. Regional dialects are generally defined by geographic boundaries. Gender differences are evident in the careful and precise language use of women versus men. Language usage varies according to the situation or context in which it is spoken. Peer group association or identification influences language usage, particularly among teenagers, often to the consternation of their parents.

Those individuals for whom English is a second language may retain vestiges of the first-learned language in using the subsequently learned language. The speech-language pathologist must determine whether the student exhibits a language disorder or a language difference. The student who has mastered the rules for a nonstandard dialect should not be considered language disordered but should be given the opportunity to learn Standard American English.

SUMMARY

In this chapter, the importance of verbal and nonverbal communication to academic and professional success has been stressed. Language has been described as a means to convey needs, thoughts, intentions, and feelings. Interindividual communication provides the avenue for controlling and directing the behavior of others. Intraindividual communication was described as being particularly useful to control and direct one's own behavior. Various aspects and levels of verbal communication were presented. Developmental aspects of receptive and expressive language acquisition were described. The guidelines were presented in such a way that they may serve as informal assessment instruments.

The nuances of nonverbal communication were described and skills for correcting errors and developing proficiency in the understanding and using of these skills were presented. Finally, the distinctions between language disorders and language differences were drawn. Chapter 3 discusses speech and language problems exhibited by special populations.

CHAPTER 3 /
SPECIAL POPULATIONS

Speech/language pathologists and teachers will find that certain groups of students are especially challenging because of their general handicaps as well as speech and language deficits. Some handicaps, such as cerebral palsy, cleft palate, and hearing impairment, require carefully planned speech and language therapy techniques when the physical impairments are severe. Learning-disabled and mentally retarded students are the largest special education groups in today's schools and most of them will receive speech and language therapy at least during the elementary grades. Behavior-disordered, visually impaired, and physically handicapped students are comparatively few in number and may not require speech or language therapy but they present unusual problems when therapy is necessary.

Schools are now assuming educational responsibility for exceptional children from 3 to 6 years of age in preschool classes throughout the United States. In many cases, a deficiency in speech and/or language is one of the reasons for classification as an exceptional student. There are also, unfortunately, some speech and/or language disorders that are acquired after normal communicative skills have been functional for some time. Some occur as a result of trauma, disease, or age-related deterioration. A brief discussion of each category may be helpful to the professional who has had limited experience with some of these special students.

CEREBRAL PALSIED

Celebral-palsied students, who have sustained injury to the central nervous system, will require special assistance in the area of communication. They present complex problems that result from the pervasive nature of their disabilities. The physical involvement is easily recognized but the less visible speech and language deficiencies may be of equal importance. The combination of physical and cognitive difficulties presents a challenge for academic achievement.

Description. The term *cerebral palsy* implies an injury to the central nervous system before, during, or after birth that interferes with the transmission of information from the brain to the motor neurons that control body movement. The location of the injury determines the parts of the body affected as well as the types of impaired movement. Faulty nerve messages may cause muscles to restrict movement (spastic type); to permit wide, uncontrolled movement (athetoid type); or to respond in a combination of abnormal movements. Injury to the cerebellum may cause incoordination and impaired balance (ataxic type) and result in abnormally slow speech.

Special Problems. Speech production may be impaired because of uneven, abnormal breathing patterns that prevent the steady, dependable airflow necessary for sound production, loudness control, and phrasing in connected speech. If the swallowing reflex is inadequate, saliva collects in the student's mouth or drools from his chin. Articulation is often difficult for these students, since lip, tongue, and jaw movements are paralyzed, weak, or poorly coordinated. Dysarthria is a common speech characteristic of cerebral palsy; impairment of the oral musculature, the laryngeal muscles, and other associated systems may cause serious feeding problems as well. Voice resonance is sometimes abnormal because of poor mobility of the velum, resulting in incomplete closure of the nasopharyngeal passage. A person with spasticity of the right side may also have a language disability due to the location of the injury in the left hemisphere of the brain, the area that has primary control of most verbal language functions. Specific language disabilities are apparent in many instances and general intellectual functioning may be below normal as well. Academic instruction may be interrupted frequently by the necessity of lengthy hospitalizations and regularly scheduled physical, occupational, and speech therapies.

Implications. Cerebral-palsied students may have mild involvement of the limbs only, may be ambulatory with several neuromuscular dysfunctions, or may have severe handicaps and be limited to a wheelchair. Although their disabilities are more visible than those of most special students, they are educated in their least restrictive environment, which is often the regular classroom. Because of multiple problems (e.g., a high percentage of the cerebral-palsied population is also mentally retarded), some students make better progress in a special class. Teachers have learned that, discounting braces, crutches, and wheelchairs, these students are as delightful as any and the satisfaction of seeing them progress is well worth any extra effort. The first concern (after medical and health) is to develop the best speech and language skills of which the student is capable. Attention should be given to breathing patterns because without a dependable airstream, there can be no shaping of sounds. The student can be taught relaxation techniques (even allowing him to lie on the floor may be helpful) as part of speech training. After the sound "ah" can be sustained on exhalation, the student is ready for some simple articulation training. The speech therapist may need to press together and release the student's lips to help him learn the motor pattern for producing [b] and [p]. Other sounds such as [f], [v], [m], [w] and [ʃ], may be produced more quickly by this manipulation method. The cerebral-palsied student often needs extra exercises to strengthen facial and jaw muscles and to increase lip and tongue mobility. Making funny faces in a mirror is fun and beneficial. Lip and throat muscles are strengthened by drinking juice through plastic tubing (from an aquarium supply store). Games for improving breath control include blowing cotton fluffs and ping-pong balls or blowing bubbles through spools dipped in soap film. Activities should be coordinated with those of the physical therapist, occupational therapist, or other special personnel serving the student. As the student struggles to improve his speech, whatever he can produce should be accepted and built upon, since it represents tremendous effort on his part. Positive reinforcement of successive approximations of the target sound will gradually shape the student's responses. It may become apparent that some students cannot gain sufficient control of the voice-producing mechanisms to be able to produce intelligible speech. In these instances, there is a range of options employing augmentative communication. The specific choice should be the system or systems most efficient and acceptable for that particular individual. It is especially important to remember the value of multidisciplinary involvement with these students. Because of the visibility of the handicap, social situations may need to be carefully structured to facilitate initial peer communication and acceptance. Expression may be limited to body language, to picture communication boards, or to mechanical or electronic augmentative devices. Even so, conversations can still take place to maintain the spirit of two-way communication and to recognize the student as an individual worth listening to.

CLEFT PALATE

The student who has or has had a cleft palate may not have defective speech. Intellectual functioning is seldom affected by this facial anomaly, so there may be no academic problems. However, some students born with cleft palates need special attention if they are to reach their full potential.

Description. The cause of a cleft of the lip and/or palate has not yet been determined, but it is known to result from a failure of the embryonic tissue to fuse normally during the first trimester of pregnancy. The incidence of cleft palate has remained about the same for several generations, so we may expect to continue to see these students in the schools. Students born with cleft palates or lips usually have had surgical repair in infancy, so there may be little visual evidence of the abnormality. There may be, however, a failure of the soft palate to completely seal the pharyngeal opening (velopharyngeal insufficiency). Some students may have a short upper lip and/or abnormal distribution of lip tissue. The palate is usually high and narrow with a residual opening in some cases, while the gum ridge often is irregular with resulting malocclusion of the teeth. Further surgery may be performed during the student's school years.

Special Problems. Velopharyngeal insufficiency *usually* results in a hypernasal voice quality and possible difficulty in building intraoral air pressure. The phonemes [b] and [p] are then produced as [m] while [d] and [t] sound like [n]. Sometimes the student can build pressure for the voiced phoneme but not the unvoiced in which case *penny* sounds like *Benny* and *time* is produced as *dime.* Other sounds may be distorted if there is poor tongue mobility. Velar closure may be imperfect, allowing air to escape through the nose and resulting in nasal vowel quality.

These students may be reluctant to speak when their voices attract negative attention. They may have poor self-concepts, especially if facial irregularities remain. Sometimes repeated surgeries delay the development of speech skills, or require the student to relearn skills after surgery. The voice may be harsh or shrill as well as hypernasal, and hearing loss is often an associated problem.

Implications. The speech/language pathologist often will consult with the medical team, reporting observations of daily speech production to help in determining the success of surgery or the need for additional procedures. Other persons in contact with the student could structure speaking situations to offer positive reinforcement. Statements such as "That's a very good answer," "What else can you tell me?" and "That's not the answer I expected but I like the way you're thinking!" draw attention to the content rather than the manner of speaking. The first objective of therapy for a student with a repaired cleft often is the development of flexibility in the lips and tongue. Mouth exercises of stretching, pursing, and twisting the lips in rapid movements are helpful and may serve to modify a constricted mouth opening. Speech habilitation for the cleft-palate student must include training in velar closure for modification of hypernasality and production of greater intraoral pressure. Encourage the student to increase the pressure by prolonging the time before air is expelled for [p], [b], [t], and [d]. Visual feedback can be provided by holding a half-inch piece of tissue at the student's mouth level to demonstrate the strength of the airstream. To reduce tension in the pharyngeal area, have the student yawn and then produce [ɔ] (aw) and [a] (ah) softly on exhalation. The therapist can then model series of words that have the probability of vowels with excessive nasality, since they follow [m] or [n]. Begin with the back vowels and move forward, maintaining the open throat as the tongue blade shifts position. Word groups could be *mall, mop, man, meal; north, notch, nail, knee;* and *maw, mud, mole, mile.* Exercises that use word pairs containing the voiced and voiceless consonant cognates are helpful to develop discrimination in production. Try pairs like *Bill–pill, bull–pull, best–pest, bale–pail,* and *door–tore, den–ten, duck–truck,* and *Dale–tail.* All these words (or appropriate pictures) can be put on 3" x 5" cards for the students to select, as in a game, and then use in an original sentence. It is important to reward the correct production of target words. Remember that many of these students must work extremely hard to control muscles and tissues that perform automatically and adequately for most of us.

HEARING IMPAIRED

Students with hearing loss experience problems in several areas of communication, although the age of the student at the onset of loss is a major determinant in the degree of interference with communication. Speech reception is impaired; speech production is usually marked by faulty articulation and perhaps by abnormal voice quality and loudness; and language skills are often delayed as well.

Description. Many hearing-impaired students have been severely impaired (hearing level of 65–85 decibels) or profoundly deaf (85 dB or above) since birth, while others have incurred significant losses subsequent to childhood diseases. The losses may be sensorineural, conductive, or mixed. Some students have congenital losses in the moderate to severe range (45–65 dB) and a few individuals have fluctuating or permanent losses of mild to moderate degree (20–45 dB) due to ear infections. Students with a mild loss would probably fail to hear the high frequency sounds—[s], [f], [θ], [ʃ], and [tʃ]—and therefore would have poor discrimination for certain words. Those with moderate losses might miss about half of a conversation held at a normal speech level and be unaware of speech at further than 8 to 10 feet in distance, unless they were visually attending. Persons with severe losses can hear conversational speech as an unintelligible mixture of faint sounds, while those with profound losses may be aware of speech inflection and phrasing but no more. These widely varying degrees of loss are classified under the term *hearing impaired.* Governmental reports indicate a prevalence of 0.5% to 0.7% of hard of hearing and deaf students in the school population.

Special Problems. Hearing-impaired children should be evaluated by an audiologist to determine how much they would benefit from use of a hearing aid. In most cases, the aid is a decided benefit and with this amplification even the profoundly deaf student with a congenital loss may develop intelligible speech. However, the hearing aid, which only amplifies, cannot solve the student's problems alone. Parents and teachers must be cognizant of the far-reaching effects of this sensory deprivation. The student can be taught to produce speech but it is meaningless without a language base. Significantly hearing-impaired children lack not only speech but also the words with which to label their perceptions. They must be taught the form of their native language and the grammar that refines it. Hearing-impaired students require instruction in many areas that appear obvious to others; their handicap eliminates many normal sources of information (e.g., overheard remarks, television programs, casual references, and a broad range of experiences). Social adjustment may be poor because the hearing-impaired student does not communicate well and does not observe accepted rules of social behavior or because others do not understand why this normal-appearing individual behaves strangely. Intellectual abilities follow the normal curve of expectation for the general population for those hearing impaired whose defect is genetic or unknown. Other hearing losses may result from central nervous system dysfunction, injury, or disease, and be associated with depressed functioning in cognition.

Implications. Special education of the hearing-impaired child should begin as soon as the loss is discovered. Parents can become excellent teachers and observers when given some suggestions, guidance, and support by speech pathologists. The speech pathologist will want to monitor the vocabulary growth and help parents to elicit first words in natural situations. Primary emphasis should be on developing spontaneous functional expression, using speech or signing according to the parents' choice. Speech should always be used with the child, even when signing. The child is continuing to learn how to use the auditory input available to her and will later demonstrate whether she can operate in the oral-aural mode. In the meantime, it has been suggested by some bioacoustical scientists that auditory stimulation could be important to the nerve receptors for further development. Connected speech directed to the child helps her to absorb the prosody (inflection, rhythm, pauses) of language, although she might not comprehend the individual words. The hearing-impaired child will profit from early enrollment in a class that is responsive to her special needs. If the loss was acquired after speech was established, the disability is less complex but still requires superior teaching and regular speech and language therapy. Care should be taken that vocabulary is taught precisely, since these students do not have the benefit of incidental auditory learning. The wise speech/language pathologist will begin articulation and voice training only after the student has become an eager and fluent speaker. The pleasure of communication should be well established before the arduous task of practicing correct production commences.

Hearing-impaired students may be integrated into the regular classroom for some or all of their instruction, or they may be taught in special classes with other similar students. Special classes are taught by certified teachers of the deaf and may employ communication systems such as sign language, finger spelling, or manual cues in combination with speech. Those students in regular classes must "speechread" by watching others' lips, faces, and body language closely while using whatever hearing is available to them. Teachers should know a few simple rules such as these: (1) Speakers should stay within 6 to 8 feet of a student who must rely on speechreading and amplification from a hearing aid; (2) the speaker should not stand between the student and the light source and should keep his face turned in the student's direction; (3) information should be presented at a rather slow speech rate and in clear, concise statements; (4) the student's comprehension should be checked frequently by visual judgment or by asking for verbal interaction during a lesson; and (5) vocabulary should be appropriate for the student's level of comprehension, with the teacher noting unknown words for future individual study. In addition, the teacher should remind the student to keep her hearing aid working properly and help other students to understand its importance so that they will respect it as well as the wearer.

LEARNING DISABLED

Learning-disabled students vary widely in the behaviors they demonstrate, but they all experience problems in organizing and utilizing new information. The learning-disabled student often experiences language problems that permeate the entire academic program. Parents and teachers are puzzled by apparent inconsistencies in performance and the student becomes discouraged when conscientious effort fails to yield successful results. Understanding and supportive families as well as skillful teaching can minimize the handicapping effect of a learning disability, but it seldom disappears completely. The underlying disorganization may continue to impede the learning process to some degree throughout the individual's life.

Description. For many years, educators had recognized the existence of students who exhibited unusual difficulties in learning, but it was not until the early 1960s that the term *learning disabled* came into general usage. Included in the U.S. Public Law 94-142 definition, *learning disabilities* are disorders in understanding and using language and disabilities in listening, thinking, speaking, reading, writing, spelling, or calculating (math). The definition includes children with perceptual handicaps, brain injury, minimal brain dysfunction, dyslexia, and developmental aphasia but excludes those whose learning problems are due to visual, hearing, or motor handicaps, mental retardation, emotional disturbance, or socioeconomic disadvantage. Prevalence is conservatively estimated to be less than 5% of the school-aged population, although some school systems identify several times that number of students.

Special Problems. Far from being a heterogeneous group, learning-disabled students vary widely in the nature and manifestation of their handicaps. Many times, a child is referred by a teacher because he is "hyperactive," "doesn't finish his work," "minds other students' business," "doesn't follow instructions," or "won't abide by classroom rules." It is only later that academic scores are found to be unusually low, even though the student appears to be capable of doing the work successfully and usually thinks he has done so. Difficulties persist even after teacher, parents, and child all realize that he is not learning as expected. An underlying language deficiency may be suspected in the student who listens attentively to a story but cannot then tell the main events in the order in which they occurred. The child who relates an experience in phrases or sentence fragments and uses baby talk beyond the appropriate age may be unable to use a more mature speech pattern. The student who has difficulty giving explanations or avoids answering questions requiring more than a brief answer may be struggling with an expressive language disorder.

Implications. Some specific activities directed toward the student's preferred style of learning may help him learn to utilize language more effectively. The multisensory approach emphasizes the use of tactile and kinesthetic cues as well as visual and auditory stimuli. A student is helped to remember the sequence and events in a story when he can point to pictures in a book or move figures from place to place on a flannelboard. Letters and numerals are learned through several senses when the symbols are touched and traced or written as well as looked at, named aloud, or sung in kindergarten rhymes. Hands-on activities are interesting and excellent educational techniques for all ages. Touching and manipulating are valuable in the shop and science lab, just as they are in the primary grades. When attention is to be directed to listening, reduce the visual distractors as much as possible and eliminate extraneous noises. If vision is the relevant modality (silent reading), provide a quiet spot or try soft background music (perhaps earphones) as a buffer. It may be helpful to plan lessons to include some physical moving about to assist the student with a high activity level to release tension in an acceptable way. Suggestions for specific language development activities can be found in Part V of this book. In addition to the traditional academic skills, social and survival communication should be emphasized. Self-monitoring techniques may be particularly important to the student to help him compensate for weaknesses. The educator who plans and executes the learning-disabled student's curriculum must consider the student's areas of strength and weakness as well as his changing needs as he grows older. It is the responsibility of the professional to adapt instructional strategies to the individual's developmental pattern and preferred style of learning and to teach him compensatory strategies in order that growth can occur, leaving failure and frustration behind.

MENTALLY RETARDED

Students who are handicapped in general intellectual functioning will almost certainly demonstrate difficulties in several areas of speech and language. They will usually begin talking at a later than average age and the development of speech skills will progress at a slower rate. Language development usually will be affected in proportion to the degree of mental impairment, although a stimulating environment, early intervention, and continued therapy will facilitate optimum growth. Many individuals identified as mentally handicapped as children respond to special education services so well that as adults they function well enough to blend into the general population.

Description. The existence of a mental handicap is usually confirmed by intellectual and behavioral testing; however, in many cases, it is the lack of normal speech that brings the child to the testing situation. Mental retardation has been defined as intellectual functioning that is significantly depressed, observed during the developmental years, and accompanied by deficits in adaptive behavior. Four levels of retardation—mild, moderate, severe, and profound—are defined in terms of scores received on tests of intellectual functioning, but a measure of adaptive behavior is a necessary component in the assessment. Most authoritative sources (federal agencies and advocacy groups) report a prevalence of 2% to 3% mentally handicapped persons in the general population of the United States.

Special Problems. Some mentally handicapped students may not be able to care for or express their own basic needs. Others may exhibit speech problems so severe that their communication efforts have limited success. When speech is intelligible, it may be socially inappropriate or inadequate. Delay in the development of language skills will be reflected in all areas of academics. Reading achievement will be depressed if the student has a restricted vocabulary, limited experiential background, or speech production problems. Social studies and science may present additional difficulties when the content moves from concrete to abstract concepts. Solving mathematical problems requires memory skills, sequencing, and the mental manipulation of symbols, all difficult for the mentally handicapped. When the retarded adult leaves school, she may have adequate vocational skills but be unable to find employment because her functional communication is not acceptable.

Implications. Mentally retarded students may follow the normal developmental pattern in the way they comprehend and use language, but they are much slower in development and will plateau at lower levels of achievement. Parents, teachers, and clinicians who are patient and persistent often can help the mentally handicapped person reach levels of language function far beyond early expectations. It is natural for humans to want to communicate; therefore, speech and language activities should be based upon desire, interaction, and results. Mentally retarded children, in particular, may refuse to participate in drill with meaningless sounds in an unresponsive environment. For the most severe, therapy may focus on helping the child shift from undifferentiated crying to a vocalization recognizable as a call for adult attention. For less severely handicapped children, beginning vocabulary should emphasize those objects and actions they find attractive. Activities built upon the real objects ball, baby, bottle, mama, puppy, and pie are of high interest and intrinsically rewarding while providing bilabial initial consonants for articulation training. For those students who exhibit basic vocabularies, expansion activities should proceed by naming familiar objects so that there is probability of many repetitions during the average day. Enhance the presentation of labels by adding descriptive words (e.g., pretty ball, big ball, blue ball, and little boy, funny boy, ugly boy, or dirty boy). Play with your voice, varying loudness, frequency, and inflection as you smile or otherwise show your involvement through facial expressions. When working with higher language levels or older students, remember to use concrete objects whenever possible and build into the lesson some physical activity or manipulation of objects and pictures. Since mentally handicapped students' speech and language development proceeds in an orderly fashion, although at a slower than normal rate, specific exercises given in other sections of this book can be adapted for their ages. A primary consideration is that speech and language should have a communicative purpose. Be an active participant in the interaction and reinforce the student for her efforts. Demonstrate the value and pleasure of communicative competence while having fun with your student!

BEHAVIOR DISORDERED

Since the enactment of Public Law 94–142, educators have made greater efforts to identify all exceptional students who are in need of special services. Some behavior-disordered students may have no speech or language problems while others have disabilities ranging from mild to severe. Students who, in past years, may have been simply labeled informally as "undisciplined" or "bad" are now given the special attention they need.

Description. The category behavior disordered includes those students whose behavior in the classroom is disruptive, demands a large proportion of teacher attention, and interrupts attention to task. These students are not remarkable because of physical appearance and evaluations do not reveal a profile that signals the likelihood of behavior problems. Unlike most other categories of exceptionality, the student may move in or out of the special group as behavior changes with time and circumstance. Although there is no predictive profile describing these students, certain conditions are frequently revealed in the behavior-disordered individual's case history. There may be evidence of unusual difficulties in infancy and preschool years, such as gastrointestinal irregularities, disturbed sleep patterns, excessive irritability, resistance to physical contact, lack of a normal emotional bond with an adult, and/or poor interaction with peers. The student may have suffered emotional trauma through parental divorce or death, physical abuse, or some other event that has greatly altered the stability of his life. There is the possibility of drug usage (prescribed or illicit) or metabolic imbalance that tends to cause deviations in normal behavior.

Special Problems. Some ramifications in the speech and language sphere may be (1) late onset of speech, (2) idiosyncratic speech patterns, (3) stream of irrelevant speech, (4) lack of speech, (5) abnormalities of loudness, pitch, or rhythm, (6) talking to self, and (7) aggressive or profane speech. Some students may be reluctant to interact verbally with peers or adults, while others interact inappropriately.

Implications. Teachers and speech pathologists should study evaluation reports carefully and perhaps confer with other professionals. It is wise to keep in mind that speech patterns reveal much about the individual's perception of the environment and his relation to it. Attempts to modify speech production and language functioning should be based on some understanding of the student's motivation and self-image. The speech pathologist can be a valuable member of the team that works with the student to expunge disorder and bring behavior into the normal range. When planning treatment strategies, observation of and listening to the student are primary concerns that continue to be important as long as the individual needs special services. Adult-student sharing of materials in play or art activities will help to establish rapport, introduce a nonthreatening subject that may overcome communication barriers, and provide a vehicle for speech and language remediation procedures. Remember that therapy is done with the student, not to the student. Remove as much stress and rigidity as possible from the adult-student relationship, since by definition this is an area of struggle for him. Appropriate communication with peers is also an important goal toward which to work; carefully structured situations for verbal interaction may improve interpersonal communication as well as speech and language skills.

VISUALLY IMPAIRED

While relatively few students are visually impaired to the degree that special education services are required, those individuals who are so impaired must cope with complex problems. In the majority of cases, there is need for speech and/or language therapy during at least part of the developmental period.

Description. A prevalence figure of approximately 0.1% of the school-aged population classified visually impaired is generally accepted by governmental funding sources. The actual number of students varies with certain disease epidemics as well as with changes in medical and educational treatment; however, the relative proportion of this exceptionality remains about the same. While it is true that any degree of diminished vision interferes with optimal functioning, only those visual deficits that cannot be corrected with lenses are included in this category. Various descriptive approaches are used but the schools usually consider the 20–200 visual acuity level as blind and corrected acuity of 20–70 or poorer as partially sighted. Other abnormalities of visual functioning, such as nystagmus, limited visual field, or lack of fusion, may justify the description of partially sighted if recommended by an ophthalmologist. Congenital visual impairment is sometimes the result of birth injury or infection, caused by a physical anomaly, or associated with other central nervous system disorders.

Special Problems. As with the hearing-impaired child, the early years are of utmost importance. Speech development is often delayed, since the child does not have the full benefit of seeing the speaker produce the sounds in words; the natural imitation of lip and mouth movements does not occur when the model is not seen. Individual sounds are often distorted by abnormal place or manner of production. A more serious although less obvious problem is the visually-impaired child's depressed ability to form concepts and to understand her environment. Much important information is not received when the visual channel is limited or nonoperative. Vocabularies are restricted by lack of experiential background and by the difficulty of comprehending certain words. There is little meaning in color words or in words describing great size or expanse (huge, gigantic, sky, moon, stars, space, etc.) for a child who can only discriminate light and dark or who can see nothing at all. Social growth is delayed due to the necessary dependence on others and to the lack of opportunity to observe others' facial expressions and body movements. These nonverbal messages provide important guides in encouraging or redirecting interpersonal exchanges.

Implications. The visually impaired student needs extra stimulation through the remaining sensory channels as soon as the visual handicap is discovered. The daily environment should be filled with sounds and efforts should be made to help the child build concepts (e.g., telephone, car, kitchen, TV, outdoors) by linking the sounds with associated events. The ring of the telephone can be followed by taking the child to the instrument, thereby locating it in space as well as providing tactile information while she hears the transmitted voice. The sounds, smells, tactile impressions, and activities of car, kitchen, or other experiences need to be woven into a rich fabric of language. Vocabulary can be developed by providing tactual contact with the referent whenever possible and by explaining new words in terms the visually handicapped can grasp. The visually impaired student needs experience with new places, new activities, and new people. Nothing will ever replace the lost sense of sight but much will be gained by a continuous effort to fully utilize the other sensory channels. The visually impaired and the hearing impaired are on opposite sides of a comprehension chasm: The visually impaired have verbal labels without associated perceptions while the hearing impaired have perceptions without verbal labels. Both groups will need assistance with language learning throughout most of their lives.

PHYSICALLY HANDICAPPED

Within the physically handicapped group are those who have orthopedic handicaps, growth irregularities, or chronic health problems. The condition may have been evident at birth, identified during the developmental years, or the result of an accident. If the speech production mechanism is not affected, the individual may have neither a speech nor a language problem. Since there are great differences of type and severity of handicap within this category, it is reasonable only to suggest that there is a higher incidence of speech and language disorders associated with all other handicapping conditions than in the normal population.

Description. To be classified as physically handicapped, the student's primary disability must relate to a physical or health condition that requires modification of the school environment to permit maximum educational development. An orthopedic handicap can result from the impaired functioning of the bones, muscles, and joints as well as from missing limbs. Students with growth irregularities, such as dwarfism, giantism, and specific syndromes, may be classified as physically handicapped and be educated in regular or special classrooms. Some chronic health problems, such as asthma, muscular dystrophy, or congenital heart defects, demand special program adjustments for the disabled students.

Special Problems. A student whose appearance is deviant lives in a different social environment from the average person. He sometimes develops needs in the affective realm that are signaled by abnormal speech or language patterns. The perception of dependency may influence the student to adopt an inappropriately childish speech or a soft, self-effacing delivery that is difficult to understand. A physically handicapped child often does not participate in many activities; therefore, the experiential foundation for building language is weak.

Implications. The school setting can provide a bridge between the physically handicapped child's world and the normal world. Fieldtrips to such places as museums, nature centers, supermarkets, shopping malls, playgrounds, farms, offices, and airports will provide material for speech and language development while expanding the student's understanding of places and people. Classrooms can become windows on the world as demonstrations by artists, musicians, sports figures, and hobbyists bring new experiences to the student. The teacher-therapist serves as a catalyst to help the student absorb information while learning to accept himself as a unique individual in a marvelously varied society. Remedial techniques for specific speech problems are presented in other chapters of this text.

Cranio-Facial Anomalies, a Special Case. In rare but tragic instances, a student may suffer gross deformity, such as absent or misplaced ears or eyes, malformation of the bony structure and tissues of the mouth and chin, or disfiguration of the face through surgery or severe burns. This student does not fit the strict definition of *physically handicapped* but is being included at this point because of the special treatment required. The student may be placed in regular or special classes for academic instruction but will almost always benefit from special attention in the areas of speech and language. Speech production may be impaired by the physical limitations of the oro-facial structure; therefore, an exchange of information between the speech pathologist and the medical team may result in better planning for the student's optimum speech capability. The student with facial disfigurement needs the same kind of supportive exposure to many social situations as the physically handicapped student. The nonthreatening therapy setting may encourage the expression of fears and resentments, thereby helping to prevent the development of communication barriers.

PRESCHOOL HANDICAPPED

The current trend is to bring children into the classroom at progressively younger ages. Federal funding has become available to provide educational services for children aged birth to 6 years who are identified as unlikely to succeed academically without early intervention. Many states or local school systems have established classes for high-risk 4-year-olds, in addition to kindergarten for all 5-year-old children.

Description. Preschool children with severe sensory handicaps (vision or hearing), severe emotional disturbance, or autism are usually identified and their educational placement may be in special categorical classes. Other children, under the age of 5 or 6, may differ noticeably from their peers and cause anxious parents to seek professional opinions. Multidisciplinary testing can reveal delays in cognitive functioning, social behavior, self-help skills, or speech and language functioning. When significant deficits are found, recommendations are made for placement in an appropriate setting designed to teach the delayed skills. Infant stimulation programs often are conducted in the baby's home or at sites other than the public schools. In-school classes that are called *noncategorical* are ones in which no label has been assigned to the child, but programming is based on observed behavioral deficits. The preschool-aged handicapped child who attends classes at school is usually from 3 to 6 years old and may be functioning at a much younger level. The handicapped child may present severe physical disabilities, depressed intellectual functioning, short attention span, hyperactivity, aggressiveness, withdrawal, inappropriate play, unintelligible speech, specific speech/language disorders, or no speech. Some children in the class may have less noticeable problems but most will benefit from speech and language stimulation activities.

Special Problems. The physically involved student may require extra space for positioning (chairs, standing table, floormat) or mobility. This student may also need
assistance with basic self-care (toileting, eating). The speech pathologist
may supervise at lunch and snack times in an attempt to develop adequate
biting, chewing, and swallowing patterns. Many times, the most noticeable
disability of the preschool handicapped child is in the speech and language
area. Sometimes the home environment has been lacking in stimulation or
may even have inhibited speech and language growth because of poor
speech models. Parents sometimes must be taught to talk to the child
appropriately and to reward early efforts of the youngster to effect changes
in the behavior of others. The child who has had little opportunity to observe
or interact outside the home and family group often exhibits significant gaps
in his vocabulary and language development. These children frequently
display social immaturity as well, which interferes with learning. Children
with certain syndromes (such as Down), will have reduced mental abilities
with little or no speech.

Implications. Most preschool-aged children enjoy and learn from a language-based
curriculum. Activities can be modified to meet the child's individual interest
level and frequent communication between home and school will make it
possible for the family to continue the same type of activities at home. It is
important that the child's caregivers be invited to share in the child's
learning experiences, since they are valuable teachers, too. The professionals can demonstrate how even severely handicapped children can participate in music and rhythm games, which often open the door to spontaneous
verbal expression. Finger plays ("Eensy Weensy Spider") or songs with
gestures ("This is the Way We Brush Our Teeth") introduce concepts that a
skillful teacher will enlarge for the more capable students. Structured play
involving the imitation of adults, other children, or animals encourages
imagination, memory, and verbalization, all basic to language growth.
Classroom demonstrations of simple food preparation and involvement in
messy paint, clay, or water projects help the child to develop many sensory
experiences upon which to build language. Daily storytime which includes
visual reinforcement of characters and actions, widens the student's world,
increases vocabulary, and provides a vehicle for indirect teaching of many
concepts. The teacher and speech pathologist will discover that sharing the
world of the preschool child can be a delightful and mutually beneficial
experience.

ACQUIRED DISORDERS

Certain disorders of communication are the result of disease or impairment
of the central nervous system that has occurred after normal speech and
language have developed. Trauma to the nervous system can happen to
persons of any age but frequently affects older individuals. They may incur
a lesion (tumor or injury) of some motor portion of the nervous system, which

then diminishes the efficiency of muscle action and may impair the speech production mechanism. Lesions in other areas of the brain may affect the ability to understand, organize, and/or use language.

Description. Speech may be impaired by dysarthria or other problems. *Dysarthria* is a general term for oral muscular involvement, which produces a variety of speech production problems. The different patterns result when different parts of the motor system are impaired. Flaccid dysarthria causes weakness of muscles throughout the oral mechanism. Hypernasality, a breathy and harsh voice, monotone, and imprecise articulation are the noticeable symptoms. In spastic dysarthria, the vocal deviations are similar but the muscles are tight instead of flaccid, producing a low-pitched, strained voice. Parkinson's disease causes a reduction of movement so that there is monotony of pitch, stress, and low volume. Speech is produced in short rushes and there may be inappropriate silences. Articulation is slurred and the voice is breathy. Other degenerative diseases in which speech becomes dysarthric are amyotrophic lateral sclerosis and Wilson's disease (a genetic, metabolic disorder). Total removal of the larynx is common in cases of cancer and of course requires the individual to learn to communicate without the natural voice. Cancer sometimes invades other tissues of the mouth or adjoining structures, resulting in surgical removal of portions of the tongue, lips, or jaw; the person then must relearn to produce intelligible speech. Apraxia is a disorder that causes the person to be uncertain as to how to position tongue and lips to produce the desired sounds and may be developmental or acquired.

Language functioning is often impaired by cerebrovascular accidents (strokes). In aphasia, the individual is handicapped by a disorder of language function which interferes with the ability to recognize and/or use words. Both apraxia and aphasia may be present after damage to the brain, which may be from disease, stroke, brain tumor, or traumatic head injury. Traumatic head injury may result from a traffic accident, sports mishap, occupational hazard, or abusive treatment, causing serious speech and/or language problems.

Special Problems. Although these conditions are typically found only among persons aged 50 or older, several problems, especially head injury, could occur in students who would continue to need educational services. Teachers and speech/language pathologists will find their resourcefulness taxed when planning programs for students who have lost previously acquired speech and language skills. These individuals, understandably, suffer great emotional shock when they discover that they can no longer communicate as adequately as before the disease or trauma (of whatever kind) to the nervous system.

Implications. The professional who is responsible for designing activities for an individual with an acquired impairment of speech and/or language should first attempt to learn as much as possible about the medical aspects. Information from the family as well as consultation with the physician will be of great help. It is important to know the premorbid level of accomplishment so that expectations for improvement are realistic. Armed with knowledge of the disability, a will for patient instruction, and a positive attitude, the professional can effect changes in the handicapped individual that will bring about improved morale and hopefully improvement of the physical symptoms.

SUMMARY

There are some similarities among the groups who present speech and/or language problems, and there are many differences. It would seem that most speech and/or language deficiencies stem from identifiable physical or neurological abnormalities. In some cases, remediation must attempt to circumvent the physical or neurological problem, while in other instances much attention should be given to enhancing experiences and building self-acceptance. Family involvement is desirable in all remediation programs, and it is crucial to the success of some.

Individuals in the groups described will differ greatly in their responses to therapy. Some will display rapid changes, some will have a lifelong need for supportive services, while others will learn to self-monitor their speech and accept their own best production. It is important to begin therapeutic procedures as soon as practicable and to continue to provide support and guidance. You are urged to seek further information concerning any of these special students who may come to you for speech or language services. It should be apparent that, although there are common needs, there are too many specific procedures to be adequately described in this small book. Two basic principles can assist in planning successful therapy procedures: respect your student as a unique human being, and have fun together!

REFLECTIONS

1. In your own words, describe *communication, speech,* and *language.* Why do you think many people confuse the three terms or use them interchangeably?
2. Briefly describe the process of speech. Be sure to include the anatomy of the speech mechanism and the physiology of speech production.
3. What is the name of the smallest unit of speech? What is the smallest meaningful unit of speech called? Describe the difference between the two terms.
4. Give some example of phonemes that are never combined in the English language.
5. In your own words, describe the following types of consonants and give two examples of each: *nasals, glides, plosives, liquids, fricatives,* and *affricates.*
6. Describe the place of articulation of the following consonants and give two examples of each: *glottals, labials, velars, alveolars, dentals,* and *palatals.*
7. Using your knowledge of the developmental sequence of phoneme acquisition, determine whether these students should be referred for professional evaluation:

age	says
6	"The wabbit wan into the fowest."
7	"My bawoon fwew up into the sky."
4	"My baby thithter thoundth like the'th hungry."
8	"Did you go to shursh on Easter Sunday?"
5	"Patrick likes to play soccer."

8. What are the four types of articulation errors? Give an example of each. Which is the most common error?
9. List the traditional sequence of correcting an articulation error. Describe each step in your own words.
10. What three aspects of voice are discussed? Why is it important for vocal quality to be appropriate to age, sex, and cultural membership?
11. What is the first rule that should be followed before attempting any correction exercises with a student who exhibits a voice disorder? Why is this rule so important?
12. Give a definition of dysfluent speech. Why is dysfluent speech so disconcerting for the listener?
13. Is a stutterer always dysfluent? Are you ever dysfluent? Examine the times when you experience dysfluency. What is happening in your environment?
14. Give an example of interindividual communication. Give an example of intraindividual communication.
15. What are the three levels of communication? Briefly define each one and give an example.
16. Give a definition of *encoding* and *decoding* as applied to the language process. How do these definitions differ from those applied to the reading process?
17. Why is it important to know the normal developmental acquisition of language? How will this knowledge be helpful to a preschool or primary-grade teacher?

18. What is the importance of a student being proficient in use of language? When framing your answer, consider academic achievement and profession.
19. Using your own words define *prosody, kinesics,* and *proxemics.* What is the value of understanding and using nonverbal language?
20. Chapter 3 discusses the special speech and language needs of special populations. What is the importance of learning about these special needs?
21. Numerous resources are available for the identification and remediation of speech disorders, language disorders, and communicative needs of special populations. Compare and contrast discussions in these sources with the information in Part I:

Johnson, D. J., & Myklebust, H. R. (1967). *Learning disabilities: Educational principles and practices.* New York: Grune & Stratton.

Langone, J., Jr. (1990). *Teaching students with mild and moderate learning problems.* Boston: Allyn and Bacon.

McCormick, L., & Schiefelbusch, R. L. (Eds.) (1990). *Early language intervention: An introduction* (2nd ed.). Columbus, OH: Charles E. Merrill.

Mercer, C. D., & Mercer, A. R. (1989). *Teaching students with learning problems* (3rd ed.). Columbus: Charles E. Merrill.

Polloway, E. A., Patton, J. R., Payne, J. S., & Payne, R. A. (1989). *Strategies for teaching learners with special needs* (4th ed.). Columbus: Charles E. Merrill.

Rakes, T. A., & Choate, J. S. (1989). *Language arts: Detecting and correcting special needs.* Boston: Allyn and Bacon.

Schulz, J. B., Carpenter, C. D., & Turnbull, A. P. (1990). *Mainstreaming exceptional students: A guide for classroom teachers* (3rd ed.). Boston: Allyn and Bacon.

Shames, G. H., & Wiig, E. H. (Eds.) (1990). *Human communication disorders: An introduction* (3rd ed.). Columbus: Charles E. Merrill.

Taylor, O. L. (1989). *Communication disorders in culturally and linguistically diverse populations.* San Diego: College-Hill Press.

Wiig, E. H. (1989). *Steps to language competence: Developing metalinguistic strategies.* New York: The Psychological Corporation.

Wiig, E. H., & Semel, E. M. (1984). *Language assessment and intervention for the learning disabled.* Columbus: Charles E. Merrill.

PART II

ARTICULATION

Articulation is speech sound production and results from coordinated/integrated movements of the lips, tongue, and jaws to shape the flow of air into sounds. The smallest unit of meaningful speech is the phoneme. Each language has specific phonemes (or speech sounds) that are combined in specific ways to form words. In the English language, phonemes are classified either as vowels or consonants and can be described as either voiced or voiceless. Vowels are produced with a relatively unrestricted flow of air in the vocal tract and are always voiced (i.e., phonation resulting from vibration of the vocal cords). Consonants are produced with a closed or constricted air passage and may be voiced or voiceless.

   In this book, the phonemic classification system used is the traditional phonemic classification, which is based on the manner of articulation and the place of articulation for consonants. Vowels are described by the highest portion of the tongue, by front-to-back positioning of the tongue, and by amount of lip rounding. Diphthongs are vowel-like sounds and are produced as a blend of two vowels within the same syllable.

CONSONANT DESCRIPTIONS

Manner of articulation refers to the degree of constriction of the vocal tract as the consonant begins or ends a syllable and usually to the type of air release. There are six generally recognized categories of manner:
1. *Plosive*—complete obstruction of the airstream followed by a quick release of the impounded air (Skills 1, 2, 3);
2. *Fricative*—narrow constriction of the vocal tract so that a hissing sound results (Skills 4, 5, 6, 7, 8);
3. *Nasal*—soft palate is lowered so that the airstream exits through the nasal cavity (Skills 9, 10, 11);
4. *Affricate*—combination of a plosive followed by a fricative (Skill 12);
5. *Liquid*—consonant with a vowel-like quality (Skill 13); and
6. *Glide*—consonant produced while gliding from one vowel position to another (Skills 14, 15, 16).

Place of articulation describes the position where the maximum constriction occurs. There are seven locations:
1. *Bilabial*—lips together (Skills 1, 9, 15);
2. *Glottal*—restriction at glottis (Skill 8);
3. *Labiodental*—lower lip to upper incisors (Skill 4);
4. *Lingua-alveolar*—tip of tongue to upper alveolar ridge (Skills 2, 6, 10, 13, 14);
5. *Linguadental*—tip of tongue to upper teeth (Skill 5);
6. *Linguapalatal*—tongue to hard palate (Skills, 12, 16); and
7. *Linguavelar*—back of tongue to soft palate (Skills 3, 11).

VOWEL DESCRIPTIONS

Front-to-back positioning of the tongue describes the location of the highest part of the tongue. The descriptors used in this classification system are front (Skill 17), back (Skill 18), and central (Skill 19). The height of the tongue is described as high, mid, or low, based on the position of the highest part of the tongue. The location of the highest part of the tongue and the tongue height are used in tandem to describe vowels. For example, [i] is described as a high front vowel and [a] is described as a low back vowel. Activities within Skills 17, 18, and 19 are purposefully arranged to begin with the high vowels, continue with the mid vowels, and end with the low vowels. Vowels are always voiced.

Chapter 4 is arranged according to manner of articulation. Correction of articulatory disorders usually follows a prescribed sequence. The strategies in this chapter present activities in the following categories: auditory discrimination, production in isolation, production in nonsense syllables and/or words, production in phrases and/or sentences, and generalization in class, at home, and on fieldtrips. In Chapter 5, strategies for detecting and correcting aberrant front, back, and central vowels are presented, beginning with the high vowels and progressing to the low vowels. The strategies for correcting difficulty with the English diphthongs are also detailed in Chapter 5.

DETECTION OF SPECIAL ARTICULATION NEEDS

Severe articulation disorders in children in the developmental period are usually identified well before the child begins formal schooling. These disorders are noticed by observant parents or possibly by child-search teams or health care professionals. Mild articulation problems, however, may not be diagnosed and treated until the child enters school. Usually screening programs will identify which children need formal evaluation. Articulation disorders that are not developmental in nature may also occur as a result of accident or injury, progressive neurological disease, or cerebrovascular accident (i.e., stroke).

Detection through Screening

Many school systems conduct systematic articulation screening programs for all kindergarten and/or first-grade students. The speech pathologist engages the child in conversation so that articulation may be observed in connected speech and notes possible articulatory disorders. Often a youngster is reluctant to speak freely with a stranger. When that happens, the speech pathologist conducts a type of structured interview in order to observe intelligibility and articulatory facility. Typically, the child's rhythm, vocal quality, and language are also noted. Students who exhibit difficulty in articulation (as well as other areas of speech) are scheduled for formal evaluation.

Detection through Formal Evaluation

Formal evaluation is much more structured and involved than the screening process. The articulation evaluation usually includes the following components:

Audiometric testing. A hearing test is administered to measure the threshold of hearing in order to determine whether sensory impairment is present. This audiological assessment indicates whether more sophisticated tests, such as tympanography are required or that hearing is adequate for the purposes of speech. A test of auditory discrimination that is designed to measure the student's ability to distinguish between phonemes is also administered.

Oral peripheral examination. The purpose of the oral peripheral examination is to evaluate the structures and functioning of the areas of the vocal tract. Structures are examined for intactness or abnormality and an assessment of their functioning is made. The structures evaluated include lips, teeth, tongue, hard palate, soft palate (velum), pharynx, nose, and mandible. In addition, diadochokinesis (rapidity of alternating movements) is observed and evaluated.

Articulation testing. Testing of articulated phonemes is possible through commercially available instruments, which enable the speech pathologist to evaluate phoneme production in isolated words and in connected discourse.

The speech pathologist is able to identify through this evaluation the position in the word where the misarticulation occurs (initial, final, or medial position) and the type of error (substitution, omission, distortion, or addition). The speech therapist also examines stimulability in order to make a prognosis and to form the basis for intervention.

CORRECTION OF ARTICULATION DISORDERS

The decision to treat a child for articulation disorders depends on a number of factors, including the child's age, degree of intelligibility of speech, level of intellectual functioning, and speech performance of the child's peers. When it has been decided to begin therapy, an individualized program is designed for the student, based on all diagnostic information. In general, therapy follows the course of acquisition training and generalization training. Acquisition training typically follows the sequence of auditory discrimination training and learning correct phoneme production in isolation, in words or nonsense syllables, and in phrases and sentences. Once the target sound has been acquired, the generalization phase begins. It is necessary for the student to demonstrate mastery of the sound in situations outside of the therapy room.

The strategies in Chapter 4 follow the recommended sequence of acquisition and generalization training in easily implemented activities. The strategies in Chapters 5 and 6 are not presented in the same sequence simply because the majority of articulation errors occur in consonant production rather than in vowel and diphthong production. The activities developed in the vowel and diphthong chapters (5 and 6) can be easily modified to follow the acquisition/generalization sequence, if appropriate. The words/phrases/sentences for practice have been carefully crafted to provide appropriate reinforcement of the target sound and to appeal to students of various ages and developmental levels. The teacher who uses these strategies should always modify the activities for the age, specific needs, and learning style of the youngster.

CHAPTER 4 /
CONSONANTS

1. PLOSIVES: Bilabial   **[p] Voiceless**   **[b] Voiced**

DETECTION Watch for one or more of these behaviors in a child 3 years or older:

- Substitutes any sound for [p], [b]
- Distorts [p], [b]
- Omits [p], [b] in any position in a word

Description. Production of [p] requires the speaker to impound a small amount of air in the oral cavity by elevating the soft palate at the posterior of the oral cavity and pressing the lips together. The sound is made when the impounded air is released with a mild explosion. Phonation does not occur. Its cognate [b] is formed in an identical manner except that phonation does occur on production.

Causation. Problems can result from organic or functional origins. Organic causes include neuromuscular dysfunction (cerebral palsy), velopharyngeal incompetence (cleft palate), or paralysis of the lips or soft palate. Functional causes may arise from inability to discriminate auditorially [p], [b]; from an inability to hear [p], [b]; or from an inability to approximate the lips.

Implications. Ninety percent of children age 3 have mastered the production of [p], [b] in the initial, final, and medial positions in words. Since this is one of the earliest sounds mastered, the child 3 or older who has not mastered this sound may also be delayed in language aspects. Children whose primary language is not English may distort [p], [b]. For example, Spanish speakers tend to conserve the amount of air expended on plosives, using only 1/4 the volume of air as native English speakers.

CORRECTION Modify these strategies for the student's learning style, needs, and age.

1. *Auditory Discrimination.* Present concrete objects whose initial sound is [p], [b]. Say the word while holding the object (*pencil, penny, Play-Doh, pony; button, ball, bike, bunny*). Say [p], [b] a number of times. Test for mastery by presenting words orally that the child must correctly identify as beginning or not beginning with [p], [b]. Progress to [p], [b] in the final and medial positions.
2. *Production in Isolation.* Sit beside the child in front of a mirror in which both of you are easily visible. Place your lips in the correct position for an initial [p], [b]. Expel the impounded air slowly and deliberately. Tell child to imitate you. If the child has difficulty, he should feel your lips and throat while you are producing [p], [b] and then his own. Light a candle and demonstrate that the

flame can be extinguished by expelling enough air while pronouncing [p], [b]. The student should extinguish the flames from varied distances.

3. *Production in Nonsense Syllables/Words.* Make up 1-syllable nonsense words with [p], [b] in the initial, final, and medial positions. The child should read them or say them after you. He should master the sound in the initial position, then the final position, and finally in the medial position.

Sample words for practice:

initial		final		medial	
[p]	[b]	[p]	[b]	[p]	[b]
puff	belt	stop	glob	apart	grubworm
pig	big	flip	bib	deposit	dabble
Pat	bat	hop	tube	supper	Flubber
parade	bold	clap	grab	ping pong	public
parasaurolophus	usurp	tab		compartment	baby

4. *Production in Phrases/Sentences.* Have the child read or repeat phrases and sentences loaded with [p], [b] words.

Sample phrases for practice:

sour pickles	baseball bat
pay bills promptly	dribble on the bib
Pink Panther footprints	bingo on B-21
pick yellow pansies	bounce the ball briskly
pick the strings of the harp	blow bubbles, Becky

Sample sentences for practice:

Polly likes her Apple computer.	The linebacker blitzed the quarterback.
Mop the floor with Super Duper.	
Patrick has dimples in his cheeks.	The baby burped after his bottle.
Peter Piper picked a peck of . . .	The ebb of the tide carried the beach ball away from the boys.

5. *Generalization.* Plan experiences for 3 settings:

In-Class Experiences. • Present an action-packed picture that can stimulate conversation about the action and that requires use of many [p], [b] words (e.g., Superman perched on a pyramid waving a pistol at the pigeons flying around his head.). • Engage the child in conversation and encourage the spontaneous use of [p], [b] words.

At-Home Experiences. • Suggest that parents and siblings reward the student for noticing and repeating [p], [b] words that occur in normal conversation. • Have the child telephone the post office and inquire about the price of an airmail stamp, the local post office budget, the bill for Express Mail.

Fieldtrip Experiences. • Visit a pizza parlor. Have the child order pepperoni with green peppers and sprinkle the pizza with parmesan cheese. • Visit a pet shop and discuss the puppies that bark, the bones that the puppies bite, the boy who puts food into their bowls, the birds eating birdseed, and the parrots and parakeets.

2. PLOSIVES: Lingua-alveolar   [t] Voiceless   [d] Voiced

DETECTION Watch for one or more of these behaviors in a child 6 years [t] or 4 years [d] or older:

- Substitutes any sound for [t], [d]
- Distorts [t], [d]
- Omits [t], [d] in any position in a word

Description. To articulate [t], [d], the speaker must impound a small amount of air in the oral cavity by elevating the tip of the tongue behind but not touching the upper teeth. The sound is made when the tongue drops to release the impounded air. Phonation occurs for production of [d] but does not occur for its cognate [t].

Causation. Problems can result from organic or functional origins. Organic causes include neuromuscular dysfunction (cerebral palsy), velopharyngeal incompetence (cleft palate), paralysis of the soft palate, or immobile tongue (Down syndrome, abnormally short frenum). Functional causes may arise from inability to discriminate auditorially [t], [d] or from an inability to hear [t], [d].

Implications. Ninety percent of children age 6 have mastered production of [t] and 90% of 4-year-olds have mastered production of [d] in the initial, final, and medial positions in words. Children whose primary language is not English may distort [t], [d]. For example, speakers for whom Spanish is a primary language tend to conserve the amount of air expended on plosives, using only 1/4 the volume of air as native English speakers.

CORRECTION Modify these strategies for the student's learning style, needs, and age.

1. *Auditory Discrimination.* Gather familiar concrete objects whose initial sound is [t], [d]. Present each object while saying its name *(toy, telephone, tacks, tambourine; doll, duck, disc, dime)*. Say [t], [d] a number of times. Test for mastery by presenting words orally which the child must correctly identify as beginning or not beginning with [t], [d]. Progress to [t], [d] in the final and medial positions.

2. *Production in Isolation.* Sit beside the child in front of a mirror in which both of you are easily visible. Place your tongue in the correct position for an initial [t], [d]. Tell the child to imitate you. Expel the impounded air slowly and deliberately. Tell child to imitate you. If the child has difficulty with tongue placement, apply a small amount of peanut butter to the alveolar ridge behind the upper front teeth with a sterile tongue depressor. (Discard the tongue depressor after 1 use.) Tell the child to feel the peanut butter with her tongue. This prompt should be gradually faded as the child learns proper tongue placement. The child may also place one hand on your throat and one hand on her own throat. There should be vibration felt for the voiced [d] and

no vibration felt for the voiceless [t]. You may also hold a small cosmetic mirror close to your lips and her lips. Breath vapor should be evident on the small mirror immediately after producing [t], [d].

3. *Production in Nonsense Syllables/Words.* Make up one-syllable nonsense words with [t], [d] in the initial, final, and medial positions. The child should read them or say them after you. She should master the sound in the initial position, then the final position, and finally in the medial position.

Sample words for practice:

initial		final		medial	
[t]	[d]	[t]	[d]	[t]	[d]
tool	dove	ticket	voted	tic-tac-toe	birthday
tummy	discover	upset	mold	glitter	paddle
terrific	dinosaur	draft	weird	butter	understand
tall	domino	gift	dared	quietly	immediate
tiger	date	belt	fooled	Humpty-Dumpty	today

4. *Production in Phrases/Sentences.* Have child read or repeat phrases and sentences loaded with [t], [d] words.

Sample phrases for practice:

tickle my fancy	dishpan hands
tempt the appetite	dog-eat-dog world
lickety-split	David Copperfield
tough toenails	dazzling duo
Tom Terrific	disgusting garbage dump

Sample sentences for practice:

Don't step on my pet worm.	Dave dropped the heavy award.
Tennis is my favorite sport.	Don't you want to dance with Howard?
Terry typed the report without mistakes.	Dial the seven-digit number, Diane.
The feisty fox terrier yipped at the intruder.	The devastating scene faded from the television screen.

5. *Generalization.* Plan experiences for 3 settings:

In-Class Experiences. • Present an action-packed picture that can stimulate conversation about the action and that requires use of many [t], [d] words. (Dozens of disco dancers trying to find space to dance on the lighted tile floor.) • Engage the child in conversation and encourage the spontaneous use of [t], [d] words.

At-Home Experiences. • Parents and siblings of the student can play the card game Concentration using pairs of cards with [t], [d] words or pictures. • Encourage the parent to label everything in the kitchen, den, or living room that contains the target sound. The child's task is to call out the labeled object whenever she looks at or passes it.

Fieldtrip Experiences. • Visit an exhibit at a local nature and science center or museum. Select 2 exhibits that are particularly interesting to the student and read the narrative aloud to her. Discuss the exhibit and name all of the concepts that contain the target sounds [t] and [d]. Write down the concepts for later discussion, review, and practice of the target sounds.

3. PLOSIVES: Linguavelar   [k] Voiceless   [g] Voiced

DETECTION Watch for one or more of these behaviors in a child 4 years or older:

- Substitutes any sound for [k], [g]
- Distorts [k], [g]
- Omits [k], [g] in any position in a word

Description. Production of [k], [g] requires the speaker to impound a small amount of air in the oral cavity by elevating the soft palate at the posterior of the oral cavity with the lips open. The sound is made when the impounded air is released with a mild explosion. Phonation does not occur for production of [k] but does occur for its cognate [g].

Causation. Problems can result from organic or functional origins. Organic causes include neuromuscular dysfunction (cerebral palsy), velopharyngeal incompetence (cleft palate), or paralysis of the lips or soft palate. Functional causes may arise from inability to discriminate auditorially [k], [g] or from an inability to hear [k], [g].

Implications. Ninety percent of children age 4 have mastered the production of [k], [g] in the initial, final, and medial positions in words. The child 4 or older who has not mastered this sound should be examined for functional defects. Children who are unable to pronounce these sounds may have a nasal vocal quality. Additionally, children whose primary language is not English may distort [k] and [g]. Spanish speakers tend to conserve the amount of air expended on plosives, using only 1/4 the volume of air as native English speakers.

CORRECTION Modify these strategies for the student's learning style, needs, and age.

1. *Auditory Discrimination.* Present concrete objects whose initial sound is [k], [g]. Say the word while holding the object (cup, coin, cat, cucumber; girl, gift, garbage can, gorilla). Say [k], [g] a number of times. Test for mastery by presenting words orally that the child must correctly identify as beginning or not beginning with [k], [g]. Progress to [k], [g] in the final and medial positions.

2. *Production in Isolation.* Sit beside the child in front of a mirror in which both of you are easily visible. Raise the back of the tongue so that it is in contact with the soft palate. A small amount of tension will cause air to be impounded. Expel the impounded air slowly and deliberately. Tell child to imitate you. If he has difficulty with placement, use a sterile disposable tongue depressor to place a small amount of peanut butter as far back on his palate as his gag reflex will allow. (Discard the tongue depressor after 1 use.) Instruct him to reach for the peanut butter with the back of his tongue. This sound is difficult to teach because it is not very visible. There should be no vibration

felt at the throat while pronouncing [k], and vibration should be felt during production of [g]. You may also hold a small cosmetic mirror close to your lips and his lips. Breath vapor should be evident on the small mirror immediately after producing [k] and [g].

3. *Production in Nonsense Syllables/Words.* Make up one-syllable nonsense words with [k], [g] in the initial, final, and medial positions. The child should read them or say them after you. She should master the sound in the initial position, then the final position, and finally in the medial position.

Sample words for practice:

initial		final		medial	
[k]	[g]	[k]	[g]	[k]	[g]
keep	gold	milk	dog	record	begin
king	gift	Jack	pig	market	forget
Kung fu	golly	poke	egg	doctor	dragon
cable	gasoline	look	frog	baker	tiger
calamity	guide	brake	hug	background	magazine

4. *Production in Phrases/Sentences.* Have the child read or repeat phrases and sentences loaded with [k], [g] words.

Sample phrases for practice:

King Kong	golden grain
queen's castle	go for the gold
combat in Africa	ugly rogue hog
nautical peacemaker	legal signature
chocolate milk	neglected beggar

Sample sentences for practice:

The broadcast confirmed the rumors.	Margaret has a guide dog.
Katie cooked too much chicken.	The ugly gang was ignorant.
Use your fork to break the bacon.	The guys gasped when the girl put
The donkey came to a complete halt.	on her batting glove.

5. *Generalization.* Plan experiences for 3 settings:

In-Class Experiences. • Present an action-packed picture that can stimulate conversation about the action and that requires use of many [k], [g] words. (A staggering drunk desperately trying to maintain his dignity in the garbage dump.) • Create a Bingo game with words containing [k] and [g]. Alternate callers so that many students, not just those who require practice, have a chance to practice the target sounds.

At-Home Experiences. • Read the Sunday comics together. Have the child explain the story or read some of the frames aloud. • Watch a televised sporting event with the child. If a VCR is available, videotape the event for future review. Note the players' names (Kareem Abdul Jabbar, Gabriela Sabatini, Boris Becker) and the plays (goal tending) that contain [k], [g]. Have the child repeat the names of the players and/or plays.

Fieldtrip Experiences. • In a department, store point out merchandise whose color contains the [k] and [g] sounds (e.g., green, gold, avocado, khaki). • At the grocery store, have the student identify food items that contain the target sounds (e.g., biscuits, eggs, garbage can). Practice the words frequently.

4. FRICATIVES: Labiodental   [f] Voiceless   [v] Voiced

DETECTION Watch for one or more of these behaviors in a child 4 years [f] or 8 years [v] or older:

- Substitutes any sound for [f], [v]
- Distorts [f], [v]
- Omits [f], [v] in any position in a word

Description. The sounds [f], [v] are continuants that are further classified as fricatives. Production of [f], [v] requires the speaker to place the upper incisors on the lower lip and release a steady stream of breath. The sounds have a frictionlike quality caused by the continuous release of air through a narrow opening. Phonation does not occur for production of [f] but does occur for production of its cognate [v].

Causation. Inability to produce the [f], [v] can result from organic or functional origins. Organic causes include neuromuscular dysfunction (cerebral palsy), absence of upper incisors, paralysis of the lower lip, or any condition that prevents proper placement of the articulators and/or a continuous stream of breath. Functional causes may result from an inability to discriminate auditorially [f], [v] or from an inability to hear [f], [v].

Implications. Ninety percent of 4-year-old children have mastered production of [f] and 90% of 8-year-old students have mastered production of [v] in the initial, final, and medial positions in words. The fricatives occur quite frequently in the English language. Correct production contributes greatly to the intelligibility of speech; conversely, incorrect production or absence of fricatives greatly impedes intelligibility of speech.

CORRECTION Modify these strategies for the student's learning style, needs, and age.

1. *Auditory Discrimination.* Auditory discrimination can usually be taught informally and indirectly in a short period of time by using minimal word pairs (i.e., words that differ in only 1 sound) in a game format. Create a bank of minimal word pairs, using the target sounds in the initial, final, and medial positions (fat: pat; four: door; fit: hit; tough: touch; roof: ruse; Jif: Jim; heifer: Heather; affair: aware; effect: elect). Present pairs of pictures that represent each of the word pairs. Instruct the child, "Show me (or point to) _____."

2. *Production in Isolation.* These sounds are two of the easiest to teach. Have the child sit across from you. Ask her to take a deep breath with her mouth open, and then exhale as if sighing. Once she can do this easily, work on proper placement of the articulators. For the [f], [v], the upper teeth are placed on the lower lip. Demonstrate that the [f] sound is created by placing the articulators in the proper position and sighing. The [v] is articulated in the same way except that phonation does occur, i.e., the motor is turned on. If

the student is having difficulty with aspiration, you can strike a safety match and ask her to blow it out with her [f], [v]. Hold the match close to the child's lips at first, being careful not to get too close. Gradually increase the distance from her lips as she becomes more proficient at aspiration.

3. *Production in Nonsense Syllables/Words.* Create lists of nonsense syllables with [f], [v] in the initial, final, and medial positions. The student should read them or say them after you. She should master the sounds in the initial position first before moving to the final and then the medial positions. Once she has mastered the sound using nonsense syllables, practice using the sounds in words.

Sample words for practice:

initial		final		medial	
[f]	[v]	[f]	[v]	[f]	[v]
four	vote	puff	five	confirm	convert
final	value	loaf	alive	before	liver
faith	veer	if	love	after	adventure
fear	volume	laugh	archive	comfort	trivial
forest	vigor	reef	dove	affect	effervescent

4. *Production in Phrases/Sentences.* Have the student read or repeat phrases and sentences loaded with [f], [v] words.

Sample phrases for practice:

ferocious forehand	vicious voter
famous loafer	forgiving victim
funny photograph	move everything
comfortable sofa	available van
four leaf clover	five villages

Sample sentences for practice:

Don't be foolish in the forest.	The victim forgave her attacker.
Steffi Graf has a great forehand.	The dove dove into the lake.
The five fell forward into the waterfall.	The wives beat the husbands in a game of Trivial Pursuit.
Forgive and forget is good advice.	Avarice is not a virtue.

5. *Generalization.* Plan experiences for 3 settings:

In-Class Experiences. • Select 5 pictures from coloring books, old reading books, or magazines that contain [f], [v] objects or actions. Have the child weave the pictures into an oral story. The story doesn't necessarily have to make sense. • Teach the child how to create acrostic poetry. Write a number of acrostic poems, using [f] and [v] words as the stems.

At-Home Experiences. • Play charades with the student. All the answers should be words and/or phrases containing [f], [v] sounds. • Sing the "Name Game" song with the child using [f], [v] names.

Fieldtrip Experiences. • Visit the public library and look up entries in the encyclopedia that start with [f], [v]. You may want to consider fireflies, volcanoes, finches, and vermin. Discuss the interesting entries with the student. Have her ask the librarian for books on her level about topics of interest.

5. FRICATIVES: Linguadental   [θ] Voiceless   [ð] Voiced

DETECTION Watch for one or more of these behaviors in a child 7 years [θ] or 8 years [ð] or older:

- Substitutes any sound for [θ], [ð]
- Distorts [θ], [ð]
- Omits [θ], [ð] in any position in a word

Description. The sounds [θ], [ð] are continuants that are further classified as fricatives. A stream of breath is emitted through a narrow opening with some pressure maintained to make the sound continuous. For these sounds, the tip of the tongue is elevated just behind the upper incisors. Phonation does not occur for production of [θ] but does occur for its cognate [ð].

Causation. Difficulty in producing [θ], [ð] can result from organic or functional causes. Organic etiologies include neuromuscular dysfunction (cerebral palsy), absence of upper incisors, complete or incomplete paralysis of the tongue, abnormally shortened lingual frenum (the small web of tissue under the front part of the tongue), or any condition that prevents proper placement of the articulators and/or a continuous stream of breath. Functional origins might include an inability to discriminate auditorially [θ], [ð] or an inability to hear [θ], [ð].

Implications. Ninety percent of 7-year-old students have mastered production of [θ] and 90% of 8-year-old students have mastered production of [ð] in the initial, final, and medial positions. Since these fricatives occur so frequently in the speech production of the English language (about 14%), correct production is essential to intelligibility of speech. Caution must be exercised, however, to avoid labeling a child *speech impaired* who displays difficulty with these sounds if he also is missing the upper front incisors.

CORRECTION Modify these strategies for the student's learning style, needs, and age.

1. *Auditory Discrimination.* Prepare lists of words that contain [θ], [ð] sounds with words mixed in that do not contain the target sounds. Ask the child to listen carefully and raise his hand every time he hears a word that contains the target sound. Since articulation of this sound is so visible, you should hide your mouth during this exercise.

2. *Production in Isolation.* Ascertain that the student is able to aspirate. If he is not, ask him to inhale, then exhale. When he can do this easily, instruct him to open his mouth slightly and raise the tip of his tongue behind his upper teeth. He should be able to produce the [θ] with a steady stream of breath and proper placement of the articulators. The [ð] requires the same steady stream of breath and placement of the articulators with the addition of phonation. Continuous production of [ð] creates a tickling sensation on the upper lip. For additional practice in proper aspiration, place a small cotton ball on the

table in front of the student. Measure how far he can move the cotton ball with each successive try. He should be able to move the cotton a bit further each session.

3. *Production in Nonsense Syllables/Words.* Create lists of nonsense syllables with [θ], [ð] in the initial, final, and medial positions. The student should read them or say them after you. He should master the sounds in the initial position first before moving to the final and then medial positions. Once he has mastered the sound using nonsense syllables, practice using the sounds in words.

Sample words for practice:

initial		final		medial	
[θ]	[ð]	[θ]	[ð]	[θ]	[ð]
thank	this	forth	smooth	birthday	bother
thick	that	both	tithe	cathedral	further
thirst	these	bath	bathe	earthquake	weather
thorn	them	cloth	clothe	monthly	mother
thug	those	mirth	soothe	Ethiopia	father

4. *Production in Phrases/Sentences.* Have the student read or repeat phrases and sentences loaded with [θ], [ð] words.

Sample phrases for practice:

thirty thousand
unthinkable thoughts
enthusiastic therapist
fourth birthday
thick cloth

their soothing grandmother
another feather
neither of them
bothering brother
clothe that heathen

Sample sentences for practice:

The thirsty man drank from the thermos.
Both filthy boys took a bath.
Nothing could interest the thin girl.
Thanks for the birthday card.

These feathers feel smooth.
Bathe before the weather changes.
The mother soothed her upset son.
Is farther or further correct?

5. *Generalization.* Plan experiences for 3 settings:

In-Class Experiences. • Have the student count from 30 to 39. • Play "I Spy." One student says, "I spy something that starts with [θ], [ð]." Students in the class must guess what the targeted object is. Each student must begin his guess with, "Is the something you spy . . . ?"

At-Home Experiences. • Sing the song "This is the way we wash the clothes, wash the clothes, wash the clothes. This is the way we wash the clothes, every Thursday morning." • Play the game Going on a Trip. Pack everything you can think of that has [θ], [ð] (e.g., toothbrush, toothpaste, washcloth, leather jacket, thick socks, things to play with, thermal underwear).

Fieldtrip Experiences. • Go to the grocery store with your child. Have the child identify food items that contain the target sounds. • Browse through a bookstore. Have the child read (or repeat after you) all the titles that contain [θ], [ð]. • While in the bookstore, point to books on the shelf and ask the student whether they are thick or thin. Notice the differences in thickness between the adult and children's books.

6. FRICATIVES: Lingua-alveolar   [s] Voiceless   [z] Voiced

DETECTION Watch for one or more of these behaviors in a child 8 years or older:

- Substitutes any sound for [s], [z]
- Distorts [s], [z]
- Omits [s], [z] in any position in a word

Description. The sounds [s], [z] are continuants that are further classified as fricatives. A stream of breath is emitted through a narrow opening with some pressure maintained to make the sound continuous. For these sounds, the tip of the tongue is elevated to the upper alveolar ridge just behind but not touching the upper incisors. Phonation does not occur for production of [s] but does occur for its cognate [z].

Causation. Difficulty in producing [s], [z] can result from organic or functional causes. Organic etiologies include neuromuscular dysfunction (cerebral palsy), absence of upper incisors, complete or incomplete paralysis of the tongue, or any condition that prevents proper placement of the articulators and/or a continuous stream of breath. Functional origins might include an inability to discriminate auditorially [s], [z] or an inability to hear [s], [z]. Tongue thrust (exerting of undue pressure on the teeth) might also be a cause of misarticulation of [s], [z]. Tongue thrust as a cause of articulation disorders is, however, a controversial issue.

Implications. Ninety percent of 8-year-old students have mastered production of [s], [z] in the initial, final, and medial positions. Since these fricatives occur so frequently in the speech production of the English language (about 14%), correct production is essential to intelligibility of speech. Often the [θ] is substituted for the [s]. This substitution is called an *interdental lisp.* When the airstream is released not from the front of the mouth but between the sides of the teeth, the resulting sound is described as "slushy." This sound distortion is called a *lateral lisp.* Caution must be exercised, however, to avoid labeling a child *speech impaired* who displays difficulty with these sounds if she also is missing the upper front incisors.

CORRECTION Modify these strategies for the student's learning style, needs, and age.

1. *Auditory Discrimination.* Use a game format to teach auditory discrimination informally and indirectly in a short period of time. Create a bank of minimal word pairs (i.e., words that differ in only 1 sound), using the target sounds in the initial, final, and medial positions (sun: bun; fat: sat; seat: sheet; sink: think; zoo: cue; peel: peace; loom: loose; maze: made; assail: avail; design: divine). Write "1" on a 3" x 5" card and "2" on another 3" x 5" card. Say the word pairs aloud while masking your lips from the student. Instruct the student to point to the "1" if the target sound was in the first word and to the "2" if the target sound was in the second word.

2. *Production in Isolation.* Ascertain that the student is able to aspirate. If she is not, ask her to inhale, then exhale. When she can do this easily, instruct her to open her lips slightly, close her teeth, and raise the tip of her tongue behind but not touching her upper teeth. She should be able to produce the [s] with a steady stream of breath and proper placement of the articulators. The [z] requires the same steady stream of breath and placement of the articulators with the addition of phonation.

3. *Production in Nonsense Syllables/Words.* Create lists of nonsense syllables with [s], [z] in the initial, final, and medial positions. The student should read them or say them after you. She should master the sounds in the initial position first before moving to the final and then medial positions. Once she has mastered the sound using nonsense syllables, practice using the sounds in words.

Sample words for practice:

initial		final		medial	
[s]	[z]	[s]	[z]	[s]	[z]
sailor	zoo	house	buzz	pencil	music
soup	zero	bus	wise	Christmas	husband
sink	xerox	face	nose	answer	visit
circus	zombie	circus	size	consider	business
swim	zoology	peace	daze	decide	newspaper

4. *Production in Phrases/Sentences.* Have the student read or repeat phrases and sentences loaded with [s], [z] words.

Sample phrases for practice:

sister sings   business newspaper
solitary dinosaur   dazzling gems
circus star   buzzing bees
toothless smile   easy-zip zipper
something simple   zippy music

Sample sentences for practice:

Patrick swims the breaststroke.   Did you xerox the zoology quiz?
That's the face of a circus clown.   What sizes are those blouses?
If you want peace, work for justice.   The newspaper reported zero
Amos decided to swim for shore.   business opportunities.
Sallie gave Sarah a surprise party.   The zebra pushed the peas with
                                       his nose.

5. *Generalization.* Plan experiences for 3 settings:

In-Class Experiences. • Have all students in the class memorize tongue twisters. (She sells seashells by the seashore.) Each student will have the opportunity to recite the memorized tongue twisters. This is a good rainy day activity.

At-Home Experiences. • Direct the parent to have the child read aloud from Dr. Seuss books. The books by Richard Scarry also contain excellent read aloud pages and are intrinsically motivating.

Fieldtrip Experiences. • Visit the public library. Locate a world atlas and have the child say the names of the countries that contain the target sounds.

7. FRICATIVES: Linguapalatal   [ʃ] Voiceless   [ʒ] Voiced

DETECTION Watch for one or more of these behaviors in a child 7 years [ʃ] or 8 years, 6 months [ʒ] or older:

- Substitutes any sound for [ʃ], [ʒ]
- Distorts [ʃ], [ʒ]
- Omits [ʃ], [ʒ] in any position in a word

Description. The sounds [ʃ], [ʒ] are continuants that are further classified as fricatives. A stream of breath is emitted through a narrow opening with some pressure maintained to make the sound continuous. For these sounds, the tip of the tongue is elevated to but does not touch the hard palate behind the alveolar ridge. Phonation does not occur for production of [ʃ] but does occur for its cognate [ʒ].

Causation. Difficulty in producing [ʃ], [ʒ] can result from organic or functional causes. Organic etiologies include neuromuscular dysfunction (cerebral palsy), complete or incomplete paralysis of the tongue, or any condition that prevents proper placement of the articulators and/or a continuous stream of breath. Functional origins might include an inability to discriminate auditorially [ʃ], [ʒ] or an inability to hear [ʃ], [ʒ].

Implications. Ninety percent of 7-year-old students have mastered production of [ʃ], and 90% of 8-1/2-year-olds have mastered [ʒ] in the initial, final, and medial positions. Correct production of [s], [z] can facilitate the mastery of [ʃ], [ʒ] because both pairs of sounds share many common features. Misarticulation of these sounds is likely to occur as [s], [z]. Since the sounds are so closely allied, substitution will not interfere significantly with intelligibility.

CORRECTION Modify these strategies for the student's learning style, needs, and age.

1. *Auditory Discrimination.* Prepare lists of words that contain [ʃ] [ʒ] sounds with words mixed in that do not contain the target sounds. Ask the child to lower his head, listen carefully, and raise his hand every time he hears a word that contains the target sound. The list of words should be organized such that the first words are grossly different and later words sound similar.

2. *Production in Isolation.* Since the most likely misarticulation is substitution [s/ʃ], [z/ʒ], aspiration is probably not a difficulty. If it is, refer to Skills 4 and 5 for appropriate instruction and practice. Proper placement of the articulators is achieved by instructing the student to place his lips in the position to make the vowel [u] and the tip of his tongue on the hard palate, then drop it down so that it is elevated but does not touch the hard palate. When the stream of air flows over the tongue, the tip of the tongue is forced slightly down from the hard palate producing these sounds. It may be beneficial to use a mirror to self-check proper lip placement.

3. *Production in Nonsense Syllables/Words.* Create lists of nonsense syllables with [ʃ], [ʒ] in the initial, final, and medial positions. The student should read them or say them after you. It is usually easier to master the sounds in the initial position first before moving to the final and then medial positions. Once the student has mastered the sound using nonsense syllables, practice using the sounds in words.

Sample words for practice:

initial		final		medial	
[ʃ]	[ʒ]	[ʃ]	[ʒ]	[ʃ]	[ʒ]
shoe		dish	garage	nation	treasure
ship		flash	mirage	emotional	measure
shape		posh	barrage	sensation	pleasure
shop		flush	triage	bashful	erosion
sugar		mesh		fisherman	intrusion

4. *Production in Phrases/Sentences.* The student will read or repeat phrases and sentences loaded with [ʃ], [ʒ] words.

Sample phrases for practice:

ship shape
flashing caution light
emotional sensation
fish dish
brash window washer
cymbals clashing

flashing explosion
coastal erosion
unwanted intrusion
treasure hunt
measuring tape
azure composition

Sample sentences for practice:

He flashed his badge and brandished his gun.
The ocean waves crashed on the beach.
His emotional condition was volatile.

She usually finished division problems rapidly.
Protect against coastal erosion.
I give my treasure with pleasure.

5. *Generalization.* Plan experiences for 3 settings:

In-Class Experiences. • Make up riddles whose answers contain the target sounds. Encourage the use of complete sentences when answering. (What does a pirate hunt for? A pirate hunts for treasure. What swims in the ocean? Fish swim in the ocean. What equipment should you use when jumping from an airplane? A parachute should always be part of your equipment when jumping from an airplane.)

At-Home Experiences. • Have parents walk through the house with the child and have him identify all objects that contain the target sounds [ʃ], [ʒ] (shirt, shoes, shoe polish, washing machine, sugar, fish, shaving cream, pencil sharpener, washcloth, sheets, measuring tape, special occasion clothes).

Fieldtrip Experiences. • Take a trip to the beach. As you walk along the beach in the early morning, discuss things associated with the ocean: seashells, ocean waves, pirate treasure, fish, sharks, the pleasurable sensations associated with the beach, the unwanted intrusion of loud motor boats, the auditory and visual sensations created by ocean waves crashing on the beach, the effects of coastal erosion, the pleasurable sensation of being on vacation.

8. FRICATIVES: Glottal   [h] Voiceless

DETECTION Watch for one or more of these behaviors in a child 4 years or older:

- Substitutes any sound for [h]
- Distorts [h]
- Omits [h] in any position in a word

Description. The sound [h] is a continuant that is further classified as a fricative. A stream of breath is emitted through a narrow opening with some pressure maintained to make the sound continuous. For this sound, the mouth is opened slightly and the tongue is behind the lower teeth. Phonation does not occur for production of [h].

Causation. Difficulty in producing [h] can result from organic or functional causes. Organic etiologies include neuromuscular dysfunction (cerebral palsy), complete or incomplete paralysis of the soft palate or tongue, velopharyngeal incompetence (cleft palate), or any condition that prevents proper placement of the articulators and/or a continuous stream of breath. Functional origins might include an inability to discriminate auditorily [h] or an inability to hear [h].

Implications. Ninety percent of 4-year-old students have mastered production of [h] in the initial and medial positions. There is no final [h] in the English language. This sound is rarely misarticulated, but it may be incorrectly omitted as a function of local dialect. It is correct to say "honor" without pronouncing [h], but it is not correct to say "humble" without pronouncing [h]. A student who commits this error should not be labeled speech impaired, but she should be taught correct pronunciation.

CORRECTION Modify these strategies for the student's learning style, needs, and age.

1. *Auditory Discrimination.* Have each child construct a paper hat. Prepare a list of words that begin with [h] and words that begin with some other consonant sound. Read the words aloud to the class. If the word begins with [h], the students should put the hats on their heads. If the word does not begin with [h], the children should remain hatless. Once the students have become proficient in this activity, create word lists with [h] in the medial position and repeat the activity.

2. *Production in Isolation.* If failure to aspirate is the problem with production of [h], give the child a small hand mirror. Ask her to open her mouth slightly, take a deep breath, and breathe onto the mirror. She should examine the mirror to see if her breath vapor is present. If further practice is needed, strike a safety match and, holding it a safe distance from the student, have her blow it out with her [h] sound. Placement of the articulators is fairly easy for this sound. The mouth is opened slightly and the tongue rests in the bottom of the oral cavity. The tongue tip should touch the lower alveolar ridge.

3. *Production in Nonsense Syllables/Words.* Create lists of nonsense syllables with [h] in the initial and medial positions. The student should read them or say them after you. She should master the sounds in the initial position first before moving to the medial position. Once she has mastered the sound using nonsense syllables, practice using the sounds in words.

Sample words for practice:

initial	final	medial
[h]	[h]	[h]
hero		aha
hand		aloha
hello		behold
high		overhead
humble		enhance
hurry		inhale
hound		cohort

4. *Production in Phrases/Sentences.* The student will read or repeat phrases and sentences loaded with [h] words.

Sample phrases for practice:

horrendous hurricane	humble Houstonians
husky homo sapiens	uninhibited hang-glider
happy animal handler	huge hippopotamus
howling Halloween ghosts	hairy hero
unhealthy inhabited house	overhauled hot rod

Sample sentences for practice:

All hail the conquering hero!

The overhang in the hotel was hideous.

Hilary exclaimed, "Ahhh," when she beheld the wondrous sight overhead.

Homo sapiens are human beings.

Hurricanes hardly ever happen in Hartford or New Hampshire or Hawaii.

5. *Generalization.* Plan experiences for 3 settings:

In-Class Experiences. • Locate Dr. Seuss books that have [h] in the title (*Green Eggs and Ham, The Cat in the Hat*). If the student is reading, have her read the books aloud. If she is not yet able to read, have her supply the appropriate [h] words, phrases, and sentences as you read the story aloud. Once the Dr. Seuss story has been read to her a number of times, she will probably have memorized the story and will be able to supply the omitted word.

At-Home Experiences. • Play the travel game. "If I were traveling to Hawaii, I would have to have my _____" (holster, hairspray, hat, panty-hose, hairbrush, hip huggers, hair dryer, history of Hawaii). Each game player repeats the basic phrase, all other objects that have been packed, and a new one for her turn. Of course, each item packed must contain the [h] sound.

Fieldtrip Experiences. • Visit a working farm. Identify farm animals and farm implements that contain the target sound (laying hen, horse, hound dog, herd of cattle, harvester, hay bailer, trailer hitch, hoe, ax handle).

9. NASALS: Bilabial   [m] Voiced

DETECTION Watch for one or more of these behaviors in a child 3 years or older:

- Substitutes any sound for [m]
- Distorts [m]
- Omits [m] in any position in a word

Description. The sound [m] is a frictionless continuant during production of which the vocal tract is completely restricted by the lips. The [m] sound is one of only three nasal sounds in the English language. The soft palate is lowered so that the airstream travels through the nasal cavity. Resonance can be felt by touching the side of the nose lightly with the fingertip. Vibration should be felt only for the nasals.

Causation. Difficulty in producing [m] can result from organic or functional causes. Organic etiologies include neuromuscular dysfunction (cerebral palsy), complete or incomplete paralysis of the soft palate or lips, velopharyngeal incompetence (cleft palate), or any condition that prevents proper placement of the articulators and/or a continuous stream of breath. Functional origins might include an inability to discriminate auditorially [m] or an inability to hear [m].

Implications. Ninety percent of 3-year-old children have mastered production of [m] in the initial, final, and medial positions. This sound is rarely misarticulated and is one of the first consonant sounds produced by infants, as in "ma-ma." The child who has difficulty with this sound is likely to have many and serious misarticulations. This sound is also a visible sound, since constriction of both lips can be easily seen.

CORRECTION Modify these strategies for the student's learning style, needs, and age.

1. *Auditory Discrimination.* Gather 10 pictures from a coloring book of things that begin with [m] and 5 pictures of things that begin with another consonant (moon, mail, mouse, mitten, money, mop, milk, monkey, match, man; heel, top, cat, bug, sandwich). On a 3" x 5" card write "m" and on another card write "m" with a line through it (like the "no smoking" signs). Show each picture while pronouncing the word. If the word begins with [m], the child should place the picture under the card with "m." If the word does not begin with [m], the child should place the picture under the "no m" card. Continue with this activity, shuffling the cards after each round, until the child has mastered auditory discrimination of [m].
2. *Production in Isolation.* Instruct the child to hum. While he is humming, have him place his fingertip lightly beside his nose. Ask him to feel the air coming through his nose. Demonstrate proper position of the lips.
3. *Production in Nonsense Syllables/Words.* Create lists of nonsense syllables with [m] in the initial, final, and medial positions. The student should read them or

say them after you. He should master the sounds in the initial position first before moving to the final and then medial positions. Once he has mastered the sound using nonsense syllables, practice using the sounds in words.

Sample words for practice:

initial	final	medial
[m]	[m]	[m]
man	broom	hammer
meat	plume	plumage
meet	dome	important
monkey	game	image
month	worm	department
Mardi Gras	room	human
March	assume	demarcate
mayonnaise	bottom	comfort
malaise	carom	undermine

4. *Production in Phrases/Sentences.* Have the student read or repeat phrases and sentences loaded with [m] words.

Sample phrases for practice:

my comfortable home	messy bedroom
majestic mountains	murky mop water
Mighty Mouse	romantic moon
mooing animal	catcher's mitt
dimly lit gameroom	vroom-vroom-vroom

Sample sentences for practice:

The Saints won the football game in the Superdome.
Imelda imitated the unassuming manner of the Mother Superior.
Have you ever seen Mighty Manfred on the Saturday morning cartoons?
Mel munched on his hamburger and drank his malted milk.
My mother and grandmother hunted in the garden mulch for fishing worms.
Marie married Martin in the garden room in a morning ceremony in May.
Momus parades the Thursday night before Mardi Gras.

5. *Generalization.* Plan experiences for 3 settings:

In-Class Experiences. • Read the book *Marvin K. Mooney, Will You Please Go Now* to the class. The title of the book is often repeated in the story. Have several children from the class take turns saying the phrase on cue. Be sure to include the child who has difficulty with the [m] sound.

At-Home Experiences. • Play "eenie meenie minee moe" with your child. (Eenie meenie minee moe, catch a tiger by his toe. If he hollers, let him go. Eenie, meenie, minee, moe.) • Locate and name all the child's toys that contain the [m] sound (marbles, He-Man, Snake Mountain, remote control car, dominoes, Monopoly game).

Fieldtrip Experiences. • Go to a shopping mall. Have the child name all the stores that contain the [m] sound. • Pick 1 aisle in the dimestore. See how many items contain the target sound. The child must say each one aloud. • At the bookstore in the shopping mall, read all the titles of children's books that contain the [m] sound. Have the child repeat the titles after you.

10. NASALS: Lingua-alveolar   [n] Voiced

DETECTION Watch for one or more of these behaviors in a child 3 years or older:

- Substitutes any sound for [n]
- Distorts [n]
- Omits [n] in any position in a word

Description. The sound [n] is a continuant that is frictionless. The [n] sound is one of only three nasal sounds in the English language. The soft palate is lowered so that the airstream travels through the nasal cavity. The vocal tract is completely constricted by the tongue at the alveolar ridge. Resonance can be felt by touching the side of the nose lightly with the fingertip. Vibration should be felt only for the nasals.

Causation. Difficulty in producing [n] can result from organic or functional causes. Organic etiologies include neuromuscular dysfunction (cerebral palsy), complete or incomplete paralysis of the soft palate or tongue, velopharyngeal incompetence (cleft palate), or any condition that prevents proper placement of the articulators and/or a continuous stream of breath. Functional origins might include an inability to discriminate auditorially [n] or an inability to hear [n].

Implications. Ninety percent of 3-year-old children have mastered production of [n] in the initial, final, and medial positions. This sound is rarely misarticulated. Indeed, most 2-year-olds have mastered "no."

CORRECTION Modify these strategies for the student's learning style, needs, and age.

1. *Auditory Discrimination.* Assemble pictures that begin and end with [n] and a few pictures of words that begin with another consonant (net, ten, can, nurse, chain, knife, spoon, nuts, moon, rain, ice-cream cone, wagon, needle, sun, clown; book, car, bowl, watch). Draw a line down the center of a piece of poster paper. Write "N" at the top of the left column and "n" at the top of the right column. Say each word while showing the picture. If the word begins with [n], the child should place the picture under the "N." If the word ends with [n], the child should place the picture under the "n." If the word does not contain the [n], the picture is placed off the poster paper.

2. *Production in Isolation.* Instruct the child to turn on her voice motor, lift the tip of her tongue, and make the air come through her nose. Instruct her to gently place her fingertips on the side of her nose and feel the air coming through it. Demonstrate proper placement of the tongue. It may be helpful to have the child look into a large mirror so that she can see proper placement of the articulators.

3. *Production in Nonsense Syllables/Words.* Create lists of nonsense syllables with [n] in the initial, final, and medial positions. The student should read them or say them after you. She should master the sounds in the initial position first

before moving to the final and then medial positions. Once she has mastered the sound using nonsense syllables, practice using the sounds in words.

Sample words for practice:

initial	final	medial
[n]	[n]	[n]
nest	rain	pencil
nose	raccoon	ransack
nothing	tune	pontoon
nickel	done	intend
nail	hen	dinosaur
gnat	loon	insect
gnome	cartoon	intonation
north	oxymoron	endoskeleton

4. *Production in Phrases/Sentences.* Have the student read or repeat phrases and sentences loaded with [n] words.

Sample phrases for practice:

rancid bacon   no money
one hundred million   dragon monkey
night manager   romantic moon
unusual animal   running antelopes
final regional game   intentional grounding

Sample sentences for practice:

Nanny noted that nothing had happened to the crane.
Never say "no" to a persistent person.
Johnny nailed his new poster near the torn one.
The hair stood up on the nape of the neck of the angry reindeer.
The poor man had no money to pay for new shoes for his 9 children.
Cynthia and Donna nursed the wilted plant back to a healthy green.
Can anyone possibly know how a nerve regenerates?

5. *Generalization.* Plan experiences for 3 settings:

In-Class Experiences. • Divide the class into 3 teams. Their task is to generate a list of 5 words each that have the [n] sound in the initial, final, and medial positions, respectively. One member of each team will act out her word and the other teams will guess her pantomime. All team members should be encouraged to guess.

At-Home Experiences. • Name each body part that contains the [n] sound (nose, knee, neck, belly button). • Sing the song "Ninety-Nine Bottles of Milk on the Wall" with your child. (Feel free to stop the song after reaching 88 bottles of milk.)

Fieldtrip Experiences. • At the grocery store have the child name all the canned vegetables that contain the [n] sound (green beans, corn, pork and beans, lima beans, spinach). • Have the child ask a cashier for 5 pennies for a nickel. • Have the child point to and name all the fruits that contain the target sound (watermelon, cantaloupe, nectarine, Granny Smith apple, tangerine, lemon, banana, Hawaiian pineapple, prune, d'anjou pears).

11. NASALS: Linguavelar   [ŋ] Voiced

DETECTION Watch for one or more of these behaviors in a child 6 years or older:

- Substitutes any sound for [ŋ].
- Distorts [ŋ].
- Omits [ŋ] in final or medial position in a word.

Description. The sound [ŋ] is a frictionless continuant. This sound does not occur in the initial position in any word in the English language. It only appears in the final and medial positions. The [ŋ] sound is one of only three nasal sounds in the English language. The soft palate is lowered so that the airstream travels through the nasal cavity. The vocal tract is completely constricted by the tongue at the soft palate. Resonance can be felt by touching the side of the nose lightly with the fingertip. Vibration should be felt at the nose only for the nasal sounds.

Causation. Difficulty in producing [ŋ] can result from organic or functional causes. Organic etiologies include neuromuscular dysfunction (cerebral palsy), complete or incomplete paralysis of the soft palate or tongue, velopharyngeal incompetence (cleft palate), or any condition that prevents proper placement of the articulators and/or a continuous stream of breath. Functional origins might include an inability to discriminate auditorially [ŋ] or an inability to hear [ŋ].

Implications. Ninety percent of 6-year-old students have mastered production of [ŋ] in the final and medial positions. This sound is more misarticulated than the other nasal sounds. It is somewhat difficult to distinguish, however, because the most common misarticulation occurs when the [ŋ] is followed by another syllable. An example would be [fɪndəz/fɪŋgŏz]. The question arises whether this is a [d/g] error or an omission of [ŋ] coupled with a [d/g] error.

CORRECTION Modify these strategies for the student's learning style, needs, and age.

1. *Auditory Discrimination.* Make a modified Bingo game. Draw a grid with 3 columns and 5 rows. At the top of the first column, write a "B" (for beginning); also write a "B" in each of the rows. At the top of the second column, write an "M" (for middle) and at the top of the third write an "E" (for end). Leave the last 2 columns blank. Call out words containing the target sound in the final and medial positions. Use the words on the next page. The student's task is to put a mark (or a bean or a rock) in the appropriate column depending on whether he hears the [ŋ] sound in the middle of the word or at the end of the word. When all 10 spaces are filled, the student calls out "Bingo!"
2. *Production in Isolation.* Instruct the child to lift the tip of his tongue to the roof of his mouth and move it backwards until he feels the "hard part" turn into the "soft

part." Now instruct him to place the back of his tongue on the soft part of his palate. Ask him to turn on his voice motor and direct the airstream through his nose. He may place his fingertips lightly aside his nose to feel the vibration.

3. *Production in Nonsense Syllables/Words.* Create lists of nonsense syllables with [ŋ] in the final and medial positions. The student should read them or say them after you. He should master the sounds in the final position first and then in the medial position. Once he has mastered the sound using nonsense syllables, practice using the sounds in words.

Sample words for practice:

initial	final	medial
[ŋ]	[ŋ	[ŋ]
	ring	drink
	hang	crank
	sung	length
	spring	Frank
	bring	ping pong
	joking	ankle
	darling	length

4. *Production in Phrases/Sentences.* The student will read or repeat phrases and sentences loaded with [ŋ] words.

Sample phrases for practice:

something ringing   cling clang
checking the length   aching feeling
thinking about everything   crank joking
bring something   cranky, lanky Frank

Sample sentences for practice:

That cranky feeling overcame Frank.
Hank was joking about anything and everything.
Spring Lee experienced a sinking feeling as she clung to the ledge.
The doorbell clanged, "Ding dong! Ding dong! Ding dong!"
A pig was making oinking noises as the boy dumped everything into the pen.

5. *Generalization.* Plan experiences for 3 settings:
In-Class Experiences. • Enlist the aid of an energetic student in the class. Give him a list of action verbs ending in *-ing* to act out for the class. As the student acts out walking, jumping, dancing, writing, and the like, the other students in the class should take turns guessing the pantomimed action. Make sure the students who have trouble with the [ŋ] sound have a turn.
At-Home Experiences. • Make two sets of [ŋ] words on 3" x 5" cards. Play the game Concentration. Each player must say the word aloud as he turns over each card.
Fieldtrip Experiences. • Take a walk in the neighborhood. Engage the child in conversation using every possible [ŋ] word. • Select a local attraction that will be interesting for you and the child to attend together. Consider such facilities as a nature center, art museum, ice rink, or story time at the library. Note all [ŋ] words for later practice when reviewing the day's events.

12. AFFRICATES: Linguapalatal   [tʃ] Voiceless   [dʒ] Voiced

DETECTION Watch for one or more of these behaviors in a child 7 years or older:

- Substitutes any sound for [tʃ], [dʒ].
- Distorts [tʃ], [dʒ].
- Omits [tʃ], [dʒ] in any position in a word.

Description. These sounds are classified as affricates. Complete closure of the vocal tract is followed by a comparatively slow release of the impounded air as the tongue sweeps along the palate backward. The sound [tʃ] is voiceless and its cognate [dʒ] is voiced.

Causation. Articulation problems can result from organic or functional origins. Organic causes include neuromuscular dysfunction (cerebral palsy), velopharyngeal incompetence (cleft palate), paralysis of the tongue or soft palate, or immobile tongue (Down syndrome, abnormally short frenum). Functional causes may arise from an inability to discriminate auditorially [tʃ], [dʒ] or from an inability to hear the sounds [tʃ], [dʒ].

Implications. Ninety percent of children age 7 have mastered production of [tʃ], [dʒ] in the initial, final, and medial positions in words. Children who have difficulty with [t], [d], [ʃ], and/or [ʒ] as separate sounds will have difficulty with the affricates.

CORRECTION Modify these strategies for the student's learning style, needs, and age.

1. *Auditory Discrimination.* Gather familiar concrete objects that contain the target sounds. Present each object while saying its name (chair, chicken; jelly bean, gentleman; patch, watch; bridge, fudge; pitcher, inchworm; refrigerator, injection). Gather other familiar concrete objects that do not contain the target sounds (ball, doll, book, pencil, dime, etc.). Say the name of each object. If the object contains the target sound, the child should hand you the object. If the object does not contain the target sound, the child hides the named object behind her back.

2. *Production in Isolation.* Sit beside the child in front of a mirror in which both of you are easily visible. Place your tongue in the correct position for an initial [t], [d]. Tell child to imitate you. Expel the impounded air slowly and deliberately while drawing the tongue backward along the palate. The lips should be open and pursed. Have the student imitate you. If the child has difficulty with tongue placement, apply a small amount of peanut butter to the alveolar ridge behind the upper front teeth with a sterile disposable tongue depressor. (Discard the tongue depressor after one use.) Tell the child to push the peanut butter with her tongue. This prompt should be gradually faded as the child learns proper tongue placement.

3. *Production in Nonsense Syllables/Words.* Make up nonsense words with [tʃ], [dʒ] in the initial, final, and medial positions. The child should read them or say them after you. She should master the sound in the initial position, then the final position, and finally in the medial position.

Sample words for practice:

initial		final		medial	
[tʃ]	[dʒ]	[tʃ]	[dʒ]	[tʃ]	[dʒ]
check	judge	fetch	refuge	achieve	adjust
church	jump	itch	shortage	inchworm	inject
chum	jest	patch	oblige	picture	challenge
choose	Jello	ouch	bridge	attachment	indigent
change	job	touch	cartilage	pitcher	Bridget
Charlie	jam	watch	cabbage	untouchable	judgment

4. *Production in Phrases/Sentences.* Have child read or repeat phrases and sentences loaded with [tʃ], [dʒ] words.

Sample phrases for practice:

scratch the itch	challenge the judgment
choose to touch	indigent gentleman
fetch the pitcher	Gerald gestured
achieve the challenge	refrigerate the fudge
chicken crunch	garbage job

Sample sentences for practice:

The wreck of the *Challenger* touched the heart of the gentleman.
Bridget became attached to the picture of the indigent underachiever.
Madge put the Jello, the jelly, and the jam in the refrigerator.
Jennifer injected the inchworm in preparation for the dissection.
There was no shortage of cribbage players among Judy, Jim, John, and Jeff.

5. *Generalization.* Plan experiences for 3 settings:

In-Class Experiences. • Present a picture of an action-packed scene that can stimulate conversation about the action and that includes many words that contain [tʃ], [dʒ] (Gentlemen stepping gingerly around the garbage in front of the refrigerator.). • Ask the student to describe how to make fudge, jelly, jam, jelly beans, and Jello.

At-Home Experiences. • Parents and siblings of the student can play a game to think of every president whose name contains [tʃ], [dʒ] sounds (George Washington, John Adams, Thomas Jefferson, James Madison, James Monroe, John Quincy Adams, Andrew Jackson, John Tyler, James K. Polk, James Buchanan, Andrew Johnson, James A. Garfield, Benjamin Harrison, Calvin Coolidge, Lyndon Johnson, Jimmy Carter). • Think of all the first names that begin with the target sounds (Chuck, Charles, Charlie, Chauncey, Chester; Gene, George, Jeffrey, Gerald, Giles, Jacob, Jason, Jennifer, Julie, Judy, John, James, Jay, Jared, Joseph, Joshua, Julian, Justin, Jesse, Joanne, Jill).

Fieldtrip Experiences. • At the local nature and science center, select an exhibit, read the narrative aloud to the child, and discuss all of the concepts that contain the target sounds. Write the words for later practice. • Check out a mythology book from the library that is on the child's level. Have her read (or read to her) myths about Jupiter, Juno, Jason, Midas and the Golden Touch, and Charon. Discuss the stories.

13. LIQUIDS: Lingua-alveolar   [l] Voiced

DETECTION Watch for one or more of these behaviors in a child 6 years or older:

- Substitutes any sound for [l]
- Distorts [l]
- Omits [l] in any position in a word

Description. The sound [l] is classified as a continuant and is further classified as a semi-vowel. Semivowels seem consonant-like or vowel-like, depending on their position in the articulatory sequence (e.g., in the word *little*, the initial [l] is considered to be a consonant, and the final [l] is considered to be a vowel). This sound is also classified a continuant because production requires a continuous, sustained stream of air. A very common substitution in youngsters who are developing speech and language is [w/l] as in "ba-woon" instead of "balloon."

Causation. Difficulty in producing [l] can result from organic or functional causes. Organic etiologies include neuromuscular dysfunction (cerebral palsy), complete or incomplete paralysis of the tongue, shortened lingual frenum, or any condition that prevents proper placement of the articulators and/or a continuous stream of breath. Functional origins might include an inability to discriminate auditorially [l], an inability to hear [l], or simply not having learned proper position of the articulators.

Implications. Ninety percent of 6-year-old students have mastered production of [l] in the initial, final, and medial positions. This sound is often misarticulated in young speakers but is very amenable to correction. The common [w/l] substitution results in speech that is somewhat unintelligible.

CORRECTION Modify these strategies for the student's learning style, needs, and age.

1. *Auditory Discrimination.* Since a [w/l] substitution is so common, it is important to determine whether the student can discriminate these 2 sounds. Write a list of words that contain [l]. In random fashion, say each word once with the correct [l] sound and once with the [w] sound substituted. Ask the student to indicate whether the [l] sound was heard in the first or second word.
2. *Production in Isolation.* Instruct the child to lift the tip of his tongue to the alveolar ridge (the gum ridge just behind the upper teeth) and apply slight pressure. The airstream flows freely around the 2 sides of the tongue. This is a voiced sound, so the voice motor should be turned on throughout production.
3. *Production in Nonsense Syllables/Words.* Create lists of nonsense syllables with [l] in the initial, final, and medial positions. The student should read them or say them after you. He should master the sounds in the initial position first, then in the final position, and then in the medial position. Once he has mastered the sound using nonsense syllables, practice using the sounds in words.

Sample words for practice:

initial	final	medial
[l]	[l]	[l]
lick	feel	follow
love	mail	believe
lead	educational	hello
late	colorful	falling
letter	hole	belong
laugh	turtle	million
length	pull	almost

4. *Production in Phrases/Sentences.* Have the student read or repeat phrases and sentences with [l] words.

Sample phrases for practice:

fall asleep	Ling Ling
follow the leader	tall tale
fly the flag, Larry	scale the hill
family belief	mail the letter
ugly stallion	stale lemonade
animal control	lazy lizard
little lollipop	large pavilion

Sample sentences for practice:

The mare's foal was destined to grow into a fearless stallion.
That dull individual monopolized the whole evening.
The tailback looked down the field at the goalpost.
Turn that helpless feeling into a hopeful feeling.
Lucille glanced at the graceful ballerina and applauded loudly.
The loyal follower listed the general's qualifications.

5. *Generalization.* Plan experiences for 3 settings:

In-Class Experiences. • Generate a list of animals whose names contain the [l] sound. You may ask the class to think of all animals whose names contain the sound. As the names are generated, write them on the board. All students should be given the opportunity to say the animal's name that interests them the most. Ask the students to tell an interesting fact or myth about the animal. Suggestions include leopard, lizard, lion, llama, alligator, antelope, eel, elk, and elephant.

At-Home Experiences. • Open the encyclopedia to "L" and flip through the pages, stopping at any item that catches the child's interest. Read the item aloud, encouraging the child to discuss the [l] entry by asking strategic questions that will require him to practice the [l] sound. • Check out from the library several of the *Zoo Books* magazines that are likely to contain articles about [l] animals. If the child is able, have him read aloud to you. Discuss the articles with him.

Fieldtrip Experiences. • At the zoo, carefully note all the animals whose names or eating preferences contain the [l] sound. Converse easily with the child so that he may practice his target sound.

14. GLIDES: Lingua-alveolar   [r] Voiced

DETECTION Watch for one or more of these behaviors in a child 6 years or older:

- Substitutes any sound for [r]
- Distorts [r]
- Omits [r] in any position in a word

Description. The sound [r] is classified as a continuant, as a semivowel, and as a glide. This sound is classified a continuant because production requires a continuous, sustained stream of air. It is also considered a semivowel, which may seem consonant-like or vowel-like, depending on the position in the articulatory sequence. Glides are so named because the sound is generated by rapid articulatory movement. Additionally, the noise is not as prominent as that in plosives and fricatives. The [w/r] substitution is one of the most common misarticulations observed.

Causation. Difficulty in producing [r] can result from organic or functional causes. Organic etiologies include neuromuscular dysfunction (cerebral palsy), complete or incomplete paralysis of the tongue, or any condition that prevents proper placement of the articulators and/or a continuous stream of breath. Functional origins might include an inability to discriminate auditorially [r], an inability to hear [r], or simply not having learned proper position of the articulators.

Implications. Ninety percent of 6-year-old students have mastered production of [r] in the initial, final, and medial positions. One of the most common substitutions in the speech of youngsters seen by speech pathologists is [w/r]. The common [w/r] substitution results in a speech defect that calls attention to itself and may cause the listener to listen to production of speech rather than the content of the communication.

CORRECTION Modify these strategies for the student's learning style, needs, and age.

1. *Auditory Discrimination.* Write a list of words that contain [r]. In no particular order, say each word once with the correct [r] sound and once with the [w] sound substituted. The [w] is selected because the [w/r] substitution is so common it is important to determine whether the student can correctly discriminate the [r] sound from the [w]. Ask the student to indicate whether the [r] sound was heard in the first or second word.

2. *Production in Isolation.* To teach correct placement of the articulators, sit in front of a wall mirror in which you are both easily visible. Begin to purse your lips but do not complete the pursing. Direct the child to imitate you. You might describe this to the student as "form your lips into a flower petal." Instruct the child to lift the tip of her tongue to the alveolar ridge (the gum ridge just behind the upper teeth) and drop it slightly so that it is not touching the alveolar ridge. The airstream flows freely around the 2 sides of the tongue.

This is a voiced sound, so the voice motor should be turned on throughout production.

3. Production in Nonsense Syllables/Words. Create lists of nonsense syllables with [r] in the initial, final, and medial positions. The student should read them or say them after you. She should master the sounds in the initial position first, then in the final position, and then in the medial position. Once she has mastered the sound using nonsense syllables, practice using the sounds in words.

Sample words for practice:

initial	final	medial
[r]	[r]	[r]
run	dinosaur	arrow
rain	filter	porridge
wreck	solar	Gerald
Robert	creator	erect
ridicule	photographer	arrange
reward	danger	hurricane
realize	teacher	around

4. *Production in Phrases/Sentences.* Have the student read or repeat phrases and sentences loaded with [r] words.

Sample phrases for practice:

narrow-minded voter

write right

arrange to avert danger

realistic thinker

terrific tennis player

Raleigh, North Carolina

Red River Revel

unrelenting crusader

solar power

instruct the teacher

Rumplestiltskin

ripe strawberries

Sample sentences for practice:

The maladroit committed an unforgivable boner.

Can you rearrange your schedule, Robin, to collect the reward money?

The ornery Tyrannosaurus Rex dinosaur was branded a rogue.

The landlord raised the rent to a ridiculous figure.

Myrtle, was it reasonable to arrest an American hero?

The wretched photographer regretted his rash argument.

The Rex parade routed through the throngs of Mardi Gras revelers.

5. *Generalization.* Plan experiences for 3 settings:

In-Class Experiences. • Write 5 [r] words on the board. Ask the children to make up a 2- or 3-sentence story incorporating all 5 words. The story may or may not make sense.

At-Home Experiences. • Play the game Scrabble with the child. Take turns making up sentences with each word as it is created on the board. • Teach the student how to play solitaire with cards. Encourage her to verbalize each move (e.g., red four on a black five, black three of clubs on red four of hearts).

Fieldtrip Experiences. • While riding in the car, read billboard advertisements, street names, and store names that contain the [r] sound. This can be made into a competitive game, if so desired, with all passengers participating.

15. GLIDES: Bilabial   [w] Voiced

DETECTION Watch for one or more of these behaviors in a child 3 years or older:

- Substitutes any sound for [w]
- Distorts [w]
- Omits [w] in any position in a word

Description. The sound [w] is classified as a continuant, a semivowel, and a glide. Production of a continuant requires a continuous, sustained stream of air. A semivowel may seem consonant-like or vowel-like, depending on position in the articulatory sequence. Glides are generated by rapid articulatory movement from one position to another and the noise is not as prominent as that in plosives and fricatives.

Causation. Difficulty in producing [w] can result from organic or functional causes. Organic etiologies include neuromuscular dysfunction (cerebral palsy), complete or incomplete paralysis of the lips, or any condition that prevents proper placement of the articulators and/or a continuous stream of breath. Functional origins might include an inability to discriminate auditorially [w], an inability to hear [w], or simply not having learned proper position of the articulators.

Implications. Ninety percent of 3-year-olds have mastered production of [w] in the initial, final, and medial positions. The [w] sound is rarely misarticulated. It is a sound frequently heard in the babbling of infants and toddlers. If the child experiences difficulty with production of [w], he is likely to have numerous and severe articulation defects.

CORRECTION Modify these strategies for the student's learning style, needs, and age.

1. *Auditory Discrimination.* Write a "W" on a 3" x 5" card. Tape a popsicle stick to the card and hand it to the child. Create several minimal pairs containing [w] (see Skill 4 for a description of minimal pairs). Ask the child to listen carefully while you say the minimal pairs. When he hears his sound, he is to raise the "W" flag (wish: dish; bind: wind; link: wink; wink: rink; wait: fate; right: white; fare: wear; teary: weary; fell: well; round: wound).

2. *Production in Isolation.* To teach correct placement of the articulators, sit with the child in front of a wall mirror in which you are both easily visible. Form your lips into a shape to blow out a flame on a candle. Have the child imitate you. Instruct the child to turn on the voice motor and keep it running throughout production of [w]. The tongue should be behind the lower teeth. The airstream flows freely over the top of the tongue. Once the starting position of the lips and tongue is achieved and the voice motor is activated, relax the lips and drop the lower jaw to complete the [w] sound.

3. *Production in Nonsense Syllables/Words.* Create lists of nonsense syllables with [w] in the initial, final, and medial positions. The child should read them or say them after you. He should master the sounds in the initial position first, then in the final position, and then in the medial position. Once he has mastered the sound using nonsense syllables, practice using the sounds in words.

Sample words for practice:

initial	final	medial
[w]	[w]	[w]
water	arrow	away
wisdom	follow	forward
winter	few	underwear
weight	cow	towel
weapon	yellow	steward
wasp	elbow	follower
Washington	crow	underway
warranty	tow	dowel

4. *Production in Phrases/Sentences.* Have the student read or repeat phrases and sentences loaded with [w] words.

Sample phrases for practice:

wanting to weigh less	how now, brown cow
forward toward victory	window washer
winging our way westward	walk on water
away with you, scallawag	wilted yellow wildflower
worthless warranty	seaworthy crew

Sample sentences for practice:

The wasp sting left a welt on Warren's elbow.
Walter knew that the wayward fellow was a coward.
Few knew that I was a follower of Howard Westworth.
Wanda Williams walked away from the bewitching window display.
Will she win Wimbledon playing with her Wilson racket?
Wouldn't it be fun to walk on water?

5. *Generalization.* Plan experiences for 3 settings:

In-Class Experiences. • Sing the song "This is the way we wash our clothes, wash our clothes, wash our clothes. This is the way we wash our clothes, so early Wednesday morning." • Teach the song "Walking in a Winter Wonderland."

At-Home Experiences. • While working in the kitchen with your child, name everything in the kitchen that contains the [w] target sound (wire whisk, wok, washcloth, Tupperware, Corningware, window, microwave oven, wall, water faucet, dishwasher, wooden spoon, Windex). • Teach your youngster the song "Where is Thumbkin?" and sing it often together. • In the garden, discuss with your child how to avoid wasp stings, ways to weed, the winding trail of ants, wind blowing the willow tree, and watering the wilted seedlings.

Fieldtrip Experiences. • At a restaurant, have the child ask, "How long will we have to wait for a table?" The child may also request a glass of water from the waiter.

16. GLIDES: Linguapalatal [j] Voiced

DETECTION Watch for one or more of these behaviors in a child 4 years or older:

- Substitutes any sound for [j]
- Distorts [j]
- Omits [j] in the initial and medial positions in a word

Description. The sound [j] is classified as a glide, continuant, and a semivowel. A glide is so named because production requires movement of the articulators from one position to another. Additionally, the noise is not as prominent as that which is produced in the articulation of plosives and fricatives. Production of a continuant requires a continuous, sustained stream of air. A semivowel seems vowel-like or consonant-like, depending on position in the articulatory sequence. This sound does not appear in the final position in the English language.

Causation. Difficulty in producing [j] can result from organic or functional causes. Organic etiologies include neuromuscular dysfunction (cerebral palsy), complete or incomplete paralysis of the tongue, or any condition that prevents proper placement of the articulators and/or a continuous stream of breath. Functional origins might include an inability to discriminate auditorially [j], an inability to hear [j], or simply not having learned proper position of the articulators.

Implications. Ninety percent of 4-year-olds have mastered production of [j] in the initial and medial positions. The [j] sound is most often misarticulated as a substitution of [j] for [l]. It is a fairly commonly occurring substitution that typically disappears without intervention as the child matures. If the child does not learn [j] from imitation and practice, however, it will be necessary to intervene.

CORRECTION Modify these strategies for the student's learning style, needs, and age.

1. *Auditory Discrimination.* Hand the child a yo-yo. Tell her that you will be saying some words that contain the [j] sound. Every time you say the [j] sound, the child is to hold up the yo-yo. Begin by saying a few words that all begin with [j] (yes, yellow, you, yet, year). Once she is accustomed to raising the yo-yo for the [j] sound, add other words that do not contain [j]. Continue until she makes no errors.

2. *Production in Isolation.* The [j] is produced with the middle of the tongue initially raised to the hard palate. The tip of the tongue is pointed downward and touches the back of the lower teeth. To teach correct placement of the articulators, sit with the child in front of a wall mirror in which you are both easily visible. Open your mouth slightly. Demonstrate the initial tongue position and ask the student to imitate you. Turn on the voice motor and keep it running throughout production of [j]. The airstream flows freely over the top of the

tongue. Once the starting position of the tongue is achieved and the voice motor is activated, drop the lower jaw to complete the [j] sound.

3. *Production in Nonsense Syllables/Words.* Create lists of nonsense syllables with [j] in the initial and medial positions. The child should read them or say them after you. She should master the sounds in the initial position first, and then in the medial position. Once she has mastered the sound using nonsense syllables, practice using the sounds in words.

Sample words for practice:

initial	final	medial
[j]	[j]	[j]
yawn		beautiful
yams		canyon
yearbook		music
yardstick		union
useful		accordion
yesterday		Paul Bunyan
young		bouillon

4. *Production in Phrases/Sentences.* Have the student read or repeat phrases and sentences loaded with [j] words.

Sample phrases for practice:

Yosemite opened yesterday.	yellow yo-yo
yelping yellow mongrel	onion yeast bread
beautiful yacht	yield to Yale
singular yardstick	buoyant accordion music

Sample sentences for practice:

The beautiful young Yolanda yodeled across the canyon.
Yes, you may have some yummy Yoplait yogurt.
The yearbook editor yawned at the absurd euphemism.
To have been clairvoyant would have made Ulysses euphoric.
Are there onions in Yugoslavia?

5. *Generalization.* Plan experiences for 3 settings:

In-Class Experiences. • Write the following list of words on the board: yes, you, yolk, yellow, lily, baby, yank, puppy, yellow, lady, yoke, penny, yo-yo, yet, pony. Read the words aloud with the class. One student will point to 2 words and another student must create a sentence using the words. Make sure the children who are working on the [j] sound have a turn to give a sentence.

At-Home Experiences. • Purchase an interesting 24-piece puzzle to put together with your child. Direct the conversation so that the youngster has ample opportunity to practice her target sound. • Walk around the yard or inside the house with your child. Give her a penny for every [j] word she produces correctly. Things you may observe include yellow flowers, yucky worms, yipping dog, wild onions, a yield sign, yourself (in the mirror), a wooden yardstick, and sheet music on the piano.

Fieldtrip Experiences. • Walk through the grocery store. Name everything you can think of that you eat that contains the [j] sound (yams, yeast bread, onions, yogurt, egg yolk).

CHAPTER 5 /
VOWELS AND DIPHTHONGS

17. FRONT VOWELS: [i] [ɪ] [e] [ɛ] [æ]

DETECTION Watch for one or more of these behaviors in a student any age if the behavior results in unintelligible speech:

- Substitution of any of the front vowels
- Distortion of any of the front vowels
- Omission of any of the front vowels

Description. Front vowels are so named because of the location of action in the front of the tongue. Height of the tongue also contributes to production of vowels. The vowel [i] is a high front vowel and the vowel [æ] is a low front vowel. The shaping of the vocal tract, primarily by movement of the tongue, lips, and lower jaw, determines which vowel is produced.

Causation. Problems can result from organic or functional origins. Organic causes include neuromuscular dysfunction (cerebral palsy), complete or partial paralysis of the tongue, or to a lesser degree complete or partial paralysis of the lips. Functional causes are associated with severe mental handicap and hearing impairment.

Implications. In a speaker whose only handicapping condition is defective speech, it is rare for that defect to be associated with incorrect vowel production. It is more common for defective speech to be associated with incorrect consonant production. The Southern speaker who pronounces [pɪn] for [pɛn] would not be considered to have defective speech but to speak a Southern dialect. Nonnative speakers of English may have to be taught American pronunciations of vowels.

CORRECTION Teach the proper tongue and lip positions for each of the front vowels, and then practice using the sample words.

1. [i] Part the lips slightly as if smiling. Raise the tongue tip as high and as forward as possible.

Sample words for practice:

Pete	meat	sweep
neat	meal	beet
peel	leap	beam
reef	peep	keep
greet	deal	dream
sweet	fleet	heat
feel	real	reap
deep	ream	keel

2. [ɪ] The lips are slightly withdrawn. The tongue tip is slightly lower and back from the [i] position.

Sample words for practice:

gift	lid	mitt
sit	did	litter
bit	kid	jitters
Jill	kiss	little
hit	hid	bitter
sitter	fitter	miss
hiss	fizz	pig
bib	milk	pin

3. [e] The lips should be slightly withdrawn and slightly more open than for [i] and [ɪ]. The tongue tip is middle height and in the front of the oral cavity.

Sample words for practice:

wait	Jake	race
paint	dame	haste
date	game	waist
rate	maim	make
name	wake	crazy
fate	gate	fame
Blake	rake	fake
face	paste	waste

4. [ɛ] The jaw is dropped slightly from the [e] position and the lips are more open and relaxed. The tongue tip is slightly lower and more back for [ɛ] than for [e].

Sample words for practice:

red	let	well
pet	dead	dress
met	jet	jell
wet	wed	fetch
bed	net	squelch
eggs	vest	belt
nest	desk	Emily
web	tent	pen

5. [æ] The jaw is dropped even more from the [ɛ] position and the lips are more open and relaxed. The tip of the tongue is at the lowest anterior position.

Sample words for practice:

Ann	cap	sap
sat	wrap	back
rat	lap	crack
Pat	map	Jack
hat	nap	cat
ax	can	fan
bag	ham	wax
tag	jam	tack

18. BACK VOWELS: [u] [ʊ] [o] [ɔ] [ɑ]

DETECTION Watch for one or more of these behaviors in a student any age if the behavior results in unintelligible speech:

- Substitution of any of the back vowels
- Distortion of any of the back vowels
- Omission of any of the back vowels

Description. Back vowels are so named because of the location of action in the back of the tongue. Height of the tongue also contributes to production of vowels. The vowel [u] is a high back vowel and the vowel [ɑ] is a low back vowel. The shaping of the vocal tract primarily by movement of the tongue, lips, and lower jaw, determines which vowel is produced.

Causation. Problems can result from organic or functional origins. Organic causes include neuromuscular dysfunction (cerebral palsy), complete or partial paralysis of the tongue, or to a lesser degree complete or partial paralysis of the lips. Functional causes are associated with severe mental handicap and hearing impairment.

Implications. In a speaker whose only handicapping condition is defective speech, it is rare for that defect to be associated with incorrect vowel production. It is more common for defective speech to be associated with incorrect consonant production. Typically, the most important factor in understanding the speech of a nonnative American when speaking English rests in the manner of pronunciation of vowels. Nonnative speakers of English may have to be taught American pronunciations of vowels.

CORRECTION Teach the proper tongue and lip positions for each of the back vowels, and then practice using the sample words.

1. [u] Pucker the lips as if giving a kiss; then open them slightly. The tongue is withdrawn and elevated in the back of the vocal tract.

Sample words for practice:

fool	boot	food
pool	hoot	rule
drool	coot	tube
Sue	tune	suit
fruit	do	lubricate
due	duel	dual
cute	mule	cube
mute	rude	ruler
suey	cure	moot

2. [ʊ] Purse the lips and open them slightly. Elevate and withdraw the back of the tongue but not as much as for [u].

Sample words for practice:

pull	hood	wool
could	wood	would

full	soot	good
cook	book	look
took	nook	rook
bush	push	hook
rookie	cookie	bookie
looker	cooker	cookbook
bull	cushion	foot

3. [o] The lips are rounded with slight tension. The tongue is withdrawn in the back of the vocal tract and is described as medium high in the oral cavity.

Sample words for practice:

rose	nose	sore
node	lone	bone
lone	coat	boat
four	soap	road
toad	rode	rope
hoe	toe	row
low	poke	folks
mow	Joan	moan
rope	roll	robe
tone	vote	doe

4. [ɔ] The jaw is dropped slightly from the [o] position and the lips are more open and relaxed. The back of the tongue is withdrawn and slightly humped but low in the oral cavity.

Sample words for practice:

Paul	fall	wall
wall	call	tall
mall	maul	awful
paw	claw	trawl
crawl	drawl	honky tonk
honk	yawn	y'all
ball	bald	donkey
want	taunt	ought
fought	taught	caught

5. [ɑ] The jaw is dropped to its most open position and the lips are open and relaxed. The tongue is withdrawn in the oral cavity and at the lowest posterior position.

Sample words for practice:

doll	hot	pot
lot	dot	cot
not	lock	jockey
hockey	dock	rock
spot	job	lob
mob	knob	drop
crop	swat	pox
bother	father	fox
box	socks	cocktail
rot	flock	soccer

19. CENTRAL VOWELS: [ɝ] [ɚ] [ʌ] [ə]

DETECTION Watch for one or more of these behaviors in a student any age if the behavior
results in unintelligible speech.

• Substitution of any of the central vowels
• Distortion of any of the central vowels
• Omission of any of the central vowels

Description. Central vowels are so named because of the location of action in the middle
of the tongue. Height of the tongue also contributes to production of vowels.
The vowel [ɝ] is a high central vowel and the vowel [ʌ] is a mid central vowel.
There are no low central vowels. The shaping of the vocal tract, primarily by
movement of the tongue, lips, and lower jaw, determines which vowel is
produced. The sounds [ɝ] and [ɚ] are essentially the same sounds. The
difference is that [ɝ] is stressed and [ɚ] is not. The same is true for the vowels
[ʌ] and [ə].

Causation. Problems can result from organic or functional origins. Organic causes
include neuromuscular dysfunction (cerebral palsy), complete or partial
paralysis of the tongue, or to a lesser degree complete or partial paralysis of
the lips. Functional causes are associated with severe mental handicap and
hearing impairment. For the vowels [ɝ] and [ɚ], difficulty with [r] will
naturally result in difficulty with these sounds.

Implications. In a speaker whose only handicapping condition is defective speech, it is
rare for that defect to be associated with incorrect vowel production. It is
more common for defective speech to be associated with incorrect consonant
production. Residents of the Northeast may have a tendency to approximate
[r] following a vowel, but speech remains intelligible. This is not considered
to be a defect of speech but rather a dialectical difference. There may also be
a tendency to add [r] following a schwa, but this is considered to be a dialect
difference, too. The late President John F. Kennedy was notable in his
pronunciation of *Cuba* as [kjubɚ].

CORRECTION Teach the proper tongue, lip, and jaw positions for each of the central
vowels, and then practice using the sample words.

1. [ɝ] Purse the lips; then withdraw the lower jaw slightly. The tongue is in a high, central
position. The phoneme [ɝ] is stressed.

Sample words for practice:

pert	mirth	jerk
nerd	herb	Herb
pearl	girl	burl
curl	furl	dirt
swirl	squirm	squirt
chirp	Bert	germ
firm	worm	yearn
learn	dearth	worth

swerve	stern	tern
conserve	hurl	Merle
turn	berm	fern

2. [ɚ] Purse the lips; then withdraw the lower jaw slightly. The tongue is in a high, central position. The phoneme [ɚ] is unstressed.

Sample words for practice:

mother	father	brother
sister	teacher	pitcher
soldier	duster	litter
blister	glitter	jitters
canter	dancer	doctor
tractor	golfer	bitter
sitter	fitter	mister
carrier	pilfer	hunter
hazard	butter	flier
enter	center	renter

3. [ʌ] This may be the easiest vowel sound to produce. Open the mouth, leaving the lips relaxed. The tongue is in a medium-high, central anterior-posterior position. The phoneme [ʌ] is stressed.

Sample words for practice:

sum	gum	hum
tub	run	rub
but	hut	cut
sun	gust	cup
bus	bust	bug
butt	jug	nut
tuck	duck	buck
bud	mud	mutt
huff	puff	cuff
under	thunder	blunder
cub	wonder	one

4. [ə] This vowel is produced in essentially the same manner as [ʌ]. The lips are relaxed and the mouth is open. The tongue is positioned in a central anterior-posterior position, slightly higher than that for [ʌ].

Sample words for practice:

above	address	alert
about	amend	assure
occur	observe	until
alone	accuse	ascend
surround	along	belong
ability	abode	abroad
anoint	accomplish	agree
again	ahead	alarm
alike	aloof	oblige
polka	scuba	Cuba
tuba	diva	lava
java	Laura	Nora

20. DIPHTHONGS: [eɪ] [oʊ] [aʊ] [ɔɪ] [aɪ]

DETECTION Watch for one or more of these behaviors in a student any age if the behavior results in unintelligible speech:

- Substitution of any of the diphthongs
- Distortion of any of the diphthongs
- Omission of any of the diphthongs

Description. Diphthongs are produced as a result of modification in the shape of the vocal tract by tongue and lip position. The vocalized breath is emitted without cessation or obstruction of the airstream. Diphthongs are blends of two vowels uttered in a single breath impulse, much like a consonant glide. The speaker can feel and hear the shift from the initial vowel sound to the ending vowel sound. Experts do not agree on which are pure diphthongs and which used to be pure vowels gliding off to weak vowels.

Causation. Problems can result from organic or functional origins. Organic causes include neuromuscular dysfunction (cerebral palsy), complete or partial paralysis of the tongue, or to a lesser degree complete or partial paralysis of the lips. Functional causes are associated with severe mental handicap and hearing impairment. Failure to pronounce diphthongs correctly may result from dialectical differences. It is incumbent upon the teacher or evaluator to determine whether a defect exists or whether the failure is due to dialect different from general American speech.

Implications. In a speaker whose only handicapping condition is defective speech, it is rare for that defect to be associated with incorrect vowel production. It is more common for defective speech to be associated with incorrect consonant production. Diphthong production is an important factor in understanding the speech of a nonnative American when speaking English. Nonnative speakers of English may have to be taught American pronunciations of diphthongs.

CORRECTION Teach the proper tongue and lip positions for each of the diphthongs, and then practice using the sample words.

1. [eɪ] This diphthong is a combination of a middle height front vowel and a high front vowel. The beginning position is the same as that for [e] and the ending position is identical to that for [ɪ] (see Skill 17 for [e] and [ɪ]).

Sample words for practice:

Aimee	pay	cake
rain	mail	pail
bait	nail	jail
gain	day	hay
may	say	way
main	sail	ale
ail	bail	play
claim	drain	plain

2. [oʊ] This diphthong is a combination of a middle height back vowel and a high back vowel. See Skill 18 for the starting position of [o] and for the ending position of [ʊ].

Sample words for practice:

row	bow	sow
sew	mow	tow
Joe	toe	hoe
go	cone	rose
vote	note	pole
toad	road	goat

3. [aʊ] This diphthong combines the low back vowel [a] and the high back vowel [ʊ]. See Skill 18 for the starting position of [a] and for the ending position of [ʊ].

Sample words for practice:

cow	wow	brown
around	pout	sound
mound	town	vow
doubt	now	gown
brow	about	round
found	noun	loud
drown	pow	clown
shout	bound	hound
pound	proud	scout

4. [ɔɪ] This diphthong is a combination of a low back vowel and a high front vowel. The starting position of [ɔ] is found in Skill 18 and the ending position for [ɪ] is in Skill 17.

Sample words for practice:

toy	coin	foil
boil	doily	hoist
moist	loyal	soil
poise	avoid	joy
coil	spoil	employ
oyster	voice	join
cloister	noise	royal
toilet	choice	point

5. [aɪ] For this diphthong, a low back vowel [a] and a high front vowel [ɪ] are combined. For positioning of the articulators, see Skill 18 [a] and Skill 17 [ɪ].

Sample words for practice:

kite	pipe	vine
tie	cry	hi
mine	pine	bite
bite	might	nine
five	fly	ripe
dime	bike	fine
dive	night	write
line	sign	divine

REFLECTIONS

1. Describe the term *intelligibility* in your own words. Compare the intelligibility of the speech of a young child with that of an adolescent. What are the major differences?

2. Listen carefully to the articulation of a "normal" three-year-old child and a "normal" eight-year-old. Target certain phonemes to focus on such as [s], [r], and [tS]. Do the two children produce these sounds with equal clarity? Why or why not? Review each of the consonant sounds noting the ages at which 90% of the children correctly pronounce the consonant phonemes.

3. What is the purpose of systemwide or campuswide screening for articulation disorders? What steps should follow for a child who does not pass the screening?

4. What is the purpose of individual evaluation for articulation errors? What are the components of a diagnostic individual evaluation? Why should the student's plan of therapy be based on diagnostic information?

5. Visit points of interest in your community such as the nature and science center, public library, art museum, university, water processing plant, recycling center, police station, post office, etc. The purpose of your visits should be to familiarize yourself with local attractions and resources. This knowledge can be woven into the fabric of the activities presented in this book. You will also be able to better plan field trips associated with generalization activities.

6. Describe the differences between acquisition and generalization of phoneme production. Is it necessary to implement activities to achieve both? Why or why not?

7. What is a phoneme? Describe how phonemes are graphically presented in this book. Why is this a good method for depicting spoken sounds? Can this system be used for transcribing languages other than English? Describe any modifications that would need to be made in order to use this system for any language.

8. Define the following terms and give at least one phonemic example: *plosive, fricative, nasal, affricate, liquid,* and *glide.* In which general category do these terms lie?

9. Define the following terms and give at least one phonemic example of each: *bilabial, glottal, labiodental, lingua-alveolar, linguadental, linguapalatal,* and *linguavelar.* In which general category do these terms lie?

10. What is the typical sequence that is addressed in teaching correct phoneme production? Describe an activity for each step in the process.

11. Teachers of children who are bilingual or of limited English proficiency may find the vowel and diphthong chapters particularly useful. Design two lessons that you could teach to this group of special-needs learners. Use the activities detailed in this unit as resources.

12. Practice several of the strategies and activities presented in this section on an adult with whom you feel comfortable. Personalize the activities and modify them to fit the needs of the "special learner."

13. Listen to audiotapes of public figures who are nonnative speakers of English such as Mikhail Gorbachev, Pope John Paul II, Ricardo Montalban. Focus on the vowel sounds. Write down selected words for further study. Transcribe those words using the International Phonetic Alphabet. How will the comparison be useful in working with students for whom English is a second (or third) language?

14. Physical and sensory defects are described in the causation sections as possible causes of articulation disorders. List several reasons why physical defects may cause articulation disorders. List several reasons why hearing loss may cause articulation disorders.

15. What is the difference between functional and organic causes of articulation disorders?

16. What is the difference between developmental and acquired disorders of articulation?

17. There are numerous resources available for the identification and remediation of articulation disorders. Compare and contrast discussions in these sources with the information in this section:

Bernthal, J. E., & Bankson, N. W. (1981). *Articulation disorders.* Englewood Cliffs, NJ: Prentice-Hall.

Boone, D. R. (1987). *Human communication and its disorders.* Englewood Cliffs, NJ: Prentice-Hall.

Locke, J. L. (1983). *Phonological acquisition and change.* New York: Academic Press.

Sander, E. (1972). When are speech sounds learned? *Journal of Speech and Hearing Disorders,* 37, 55–63.

Shames, G. H., & Wiig, E. H. (Eds.) (1990). *Human communication disorders: An introduction.* (3rd ed.). Columbus, OH: Charles E. Merrill.

Shriberg, L. D. (1980). Developmental phonological disorders. In T. J. Hixon, J. H. Saxman, and L. D. Shriberg (Eds.), *Introduction to communication disorders.* Englewood Cliffs, NJ: Prentice-Hall.

Sommers, R. K. (1983). *Articulation disorders.* Englewood Cliffs, NJ: Prentice-Hall.

Stemple, J.C., & Holcomb, B. J. (1988). Effective voice and articulation. Columbus, OH: Charles E. Merrill.

Van Riper, C. (1978). *Speech correction: Principles and methods* (6th ed.). Englewood Cliffs, NJ: Prentice-Hall.

Van Riper, C., & Emerick, L. (1984). *Speech correction: An introduction to speech pathology and audiology* (7th ed.). Englewood Cliffs, NJ: Prentice-Hall.

PART III

VOICE

One way of expressing thought or language is through oral speech, which is made possible by vocal production. The production of speech is a peculiarly human attribute. No other member of the animal kingdom can produce sounds with such range and complexity. The vocal folds are the main sound producers. These two bands of tissue stretch across the larynx (or voice box). When breath is exhaled, the vocal folds relax to form a V-shaped opening to let the air through. To produce sound, the vocal folds are brought together, the expelled air from the lungs sets the tightened folds in vibration, and voice results.

The vocal mechanism is well organized; most people use their lungs, vocal folds, laryngeal muscles, and speech articulators (jaw, lips, tongue) without thinking about them. They unconsciously adjust the vocal mechanism to produce a voice that is similar to those of others in the social group. As beauty lies in the eye of the beholder, so normal voice lies in the ear of the listener. Voices vary in pitch, loudness, quality, and other less definable aspects and listeners react to them according to their own individual standards.

Occasionally, a voice will vary so noticeably from the accepted norm that it will be regarded as disordered. There are three aspects to consider in voice disorders: (1) the acoustic element that is heard; (2) the function of the mechanism that produces the deviation; and (3) the condition of the larynx.

Voice is considered to be defective if the vocal pitch is inappropriate for the age and sex of the speaker. Chapter 6 discusses pitch that is too high, too low, or almost a monotone. Possible causes are mentioned, including disease, vocal nodules, or voice abuse, along with suggestions for alteration of distracting and possibly damaging vocal pitch.

Loudness is considered a disorder if the level of volume is inappropriate for the circumstance, inadequate for communication, or unpleasant for the listener. Chapter 7 considers the problem of abnormal intensity or loudness in the speaking voice. It should be noted that young children often have not learned to speak at the loudness level accepted as normal by their social group. This is not considered to be a vocal deviancy in a child under 7 years of age, but investigation of the cause of this unusual behavior should be recommended. Intervention of another kind may be needed, such as medical or psychological evaluation or hearing habilitation.

Voice quality deviations are the most common and the most complex of the vocal problems. Chapter 8 includes a view of deviations associated with sound generation, the hoarse and the breathy voice, as well as consideration of resonance problems. Hypernasality, one of the most common of these, may develop because of physiological or environmental factors.

It is imperative to determine the cause of a defective voice and the speech/language pathologist must refer the deviant speaker for a medical examination before going further. After the examination, if the physician recommends voice therapy, the speech pathologist should consult frequently with the medical specialists as therapy progresses. Improper voice usage could exacerbate vocal nodules or other pathological conditions.

Vocal rehabilitation can alleviate or eliminate vocal abuse and misuse by retraining the speaker's habits. Change may also be effected by examining etiological factors that have caused or maintain the voice defect. If surgery is performed on any part of the voice-producing mechanism, the speech pathologist can assist the student in adjusting to the changes that have occurred. Attention to vocal production may allow the speaker to present to the world a more appropriate and pleasant voice, which will better reflect the person within.

CHAPTER 6 /
PITCH

21. TOO HIGH OR TOO LOW PITCH

DETECTION Watch for one or more of these behaviors in a school-aged student:

- Pitch too high for age, sex, and/or cultural expectations
- Pitch too low for age, sex, and/or cultural expectations

Description. Frequency is determined by amount of tension of the vibrating vocal folds, the mass of the vibrator (i.e., vocal folds), and the length of the vocal folds. The pitch of the voice is raised when the vocal folds are elongated because the tension is increased and the mass of the vocal folds at all points along their length is reduced. Although a shorter vibrator usually produces a higher frequency sound, the increased tension and reduced mass counteract the elongation and result in a higher frequency.

Causation. Problems can result from organic or functional origins. Organic causes include neuromuscular dysfunction (cerebral palsy), paralysis of the vocal folds, trauma or surgical modification, poor physical health, debilitating diseases and conditions, tumors, polyps, vocal nodules, edema, and laryngeal web. Functional causes may arise from vocal abuse (e.g., constant clearing of the throat, smoking of tobacco products) and/or vocal misuse (e.g., speaking at the top or bottom of the pitch range, screaming, yelling in the wrong pitch range) and may subsequently result in nodules.

Implications. Vocal pitch that is too high or too low calls attention to the manner of speaking rather than the content of speech. This probably will result in inadequate communication. For a school-aged child, psychological development may be impaired because of the reaction of fellow students. It is quite normal, however, for adolescent males to experience transient periods of too high pitch during puberty. For adults, the implication is serious in that attaining or advancing in the chosen profession may not be possible if oral communication is required as a part of the usual workday. (Rare is the profession that does not require daily oral communication.) *Always obtain medical clearance before attempting to train or retrain pitch.*

CORRECTION After obtaining medical clearance, modify these strategies for the student's learning style, needs, and age.

1. *Optimum Pitch.* Determine optimum pitch by having the student intone as low as he can and then raise the level 1 step at a time until falsetto is reached. It is helpful to use a piano or pitch pipe to match pitch levels with those of the musical scale in finding total pitch range. The optimum pitch for that student considering age and physical development is about 1/4 to 1/3 above

the lowest level within his pitch range. If 15 levels are produced during this exercise, optimum pitch is probably 4–5 levels above the lowest level. Use a piano to identify that level for the student and as a target level for approximation.

2. *Pitch Imitation.* Set up a tape recorder with a built-in microphone to record the following exercise. Instruct the student that you will produce a tone that he is to imitate immediately after you. Start by producing a low tone and go up the musical scale. Repeat this several times until the student can fairly easily approximate your tone. Once mastery of this activity is achieved, continue with the imitation exercise, producing random tones for the student to imitate. Gauge the number of tones and the range of tones to the student's performance. If he is relatively successful, the exercise can be prolonged. If he is struggling, limit the number and range of tones in the exercise. End the exercise on a successful response. Play back the tape for reinforcement for the student.

3. *Vowel Play.* Practice with selected vowel sounds [i, e, o, œ, a] to give a more meaningful flavor to pitch alterations. Say the vowel sounds aloud. Point out to the student that the sounds progress from higher frequency sounds to lower frequency sounds. Instruct the student to place his fingertips lightly on his larynx (Adam's apple). Tell him to feel with his fingertips and also with the inside of his throat the variation as the sounds change from a higher to a lower pitch. He should concentrate on how each vowel sound feels externally and internally. It is advisable to go from high to low if the objective is to lower the pitch. If the student's difficulty is pitch that is too low, then he should perform the exercise beginning with the low-pitched vowels and progressing to the higher-pitched sounds. Once the student has mastered and feels comfortable with isolated vowel sounds, practice the same vowels embedded in single syllable words.

Sample words for practice:

lead	laid	load	lad	lot
me	may	Moe	mad	mock
team	tame	tome	tam	Tom
real	rail	role	rat	rock
feet	gate	gnome	Dad	top

Sample sentences for practice:

Pete may throw that rock.	Stop that old gray jeep.
Green grapes grow bad spots.	Dom had sown grape seeds.
She hates coke that rots.	Tom had grown eight feet.
We may rope that fox.	

4. *Animal Talk.* Take a trip to the zoo. As you walk around the compound, listen to the monkeys chatter, the lions roar, the seals bark, the peacocks squeal, and the elephants trumpet. In concert with the child, imitate the animals' "talk," focusing on the frequency of the sound. Guide the child to select the pitch of animal that sounds most pleasant and that he should sound like.

22. MONOTONE PITCH

DETECTION Watch for students who display:

- Very little change of pitch
- Little variation in loudness level
- Little emotional affect in speech
- Poor intelligibility

Description. A student's voice is sometimes so lacking in melody, inflection, and variation of intensity that it approaches a monotone. This type of speech delivery affects the listener negatively and becomes a barrier to communication. Characters who speak in a monotone occasionally appear in TV programs or advertising commercials and are viewed as comical because their vocal behavior fails to reflect the message of their words or the events transpiring around them. In real life, however, they are not comical but sadly ineffective speakers.

Causation. The speech pathologist will necessarily require that the student be seen by an otolaryngologist. That medical report will indicate if physical factors are causing the monotone pitch. It is possible that the vocal mechanism is structurally stiff and unresponsive. There may be a lack of flexibility of the muscles subsequent to infectious disease or due to general neuromuscular impairment. The peripheral nerves controlling phonation may have been damaged so that monopitch is the only pattern available to the individual. However, in many cases, the monotone pitch cannot be traced to a structural cause. Some persons exhibit general hypotension or low physical/neural vitality. This is sometimes a familial characteristic and at other times the product of a debilitating illness. The lack of vitality in other cases seems due to intellectual insensitivity. A monopitch may have been deliberately chosen by the speaker as an indication of sophistication or sexual attractiveness. Conversely, the environment may have influenced the speaker unconsciously to develop feelings of inferiority or self-consciousness. Some families school themselves to repress emotion in speech as well as in behavior, and a flat delivery lacking in affect is normal for them. The individual could have developed a monotone delivery in an attempt to attract as little attention as possible. The monotone voice serves as a convenient masking device and shields the speaker from revealing her emotional feelings.

Implications. Monotone speakers will find that they are not successful communicators; therefore, many vocations will not be appropriate for them. Social interaction will suffer because of their peculiar speech and they may find themselves to be the objects of unwanted attention from others. Since one's voice is closely entwined with one's emotions, therapy may involve helping the student to change her mental outlook before lasting shifts in vocal patterning can occur.

CORRECTION After obtaining medical clearance, modify these strategies according to the student's learning style, needs, and age.

1. *Music Time.* Have the student match her voice to notes from a piano or other musical instrument from the bottom to top of an octave that contains her normal pitch. Begin by going note to note, followed by skipping notes,and then from lowest to highest notes and back.
2. *Bouncing Ball.* Use visual cues by preparing posters that depict a ball rolling along a flat line, falling down at a break in the line, and bouncing up to different heights above the line. Ask the student to vocalize with the same single syllable ("ah," "me," "red"), elevating or lowering the voice pitch to match the visual pattern.
3. *Bouncing Words.* Ask the student to use short sentences, producing each syllable in relation to the position of the bouncing ball. Have prepared sentences such as:
    > Give the dog a bone.
    > He found a dollar.
    > I like my new voice.

    Stand beside the chart and assist the student by raising your hand in the air to the indicated levels.
4. *Up or Down?* Write short phrases on 3" x 5" cards, indicating by the placement of the words the desired pitch of the voice. The student will select a card and reproduce the vocal pattern.

(1)	UP!	(2) STEP	
	STEP		DOWN!
(3)	NO?	(4) OH	
	OH		NO.
(5)	WHOM?	(6) FOR	
	FOR		US.

5. *Say It Again.* Write a short sentence on a 3" x 5" card and ask the student to read the sentence several times, accenting a different word each time it is read. Discuss the difference in meaning when the accent is changed. Be sure that the student does not substitute a change in loudness for a change in pitch.
6. *Exclaim!* Write sentences with emotional content on cards for the student to read with vivid and genuine expression, as if she really means it. Some sample sentences are:
    > Frankly, my dear, I couldn't care less!
    > But I love you!
    > The house is on fire!
    > There's been an accident!
    > Have a good day!
    > He makes me furious!
    > The baby is very sick!
    > We saw the funniest movie ever last night!

CHAPTER 7 /
INTENSITY

23. TOO LOUD VOICE

DETECTION This is a problem if a student over 6 years of age displays:

- Unpleasant, piercing voice
- Conversational volume louder than other speakers
- Speech volume inappropriate for the situation

Description. Some students come to therapy not because of personal dissatisfaction with their manner of speaking but because significant others in their lives are concerned for them. These students usually do not feel that they have a speech problem of any kind and may therefore be somewhat resistant to therapy. Some individuals habitually speak in loud and discordant tones, which makes listening unpleasant and actually uncomfortable. The excessive loudness may be accompanied by a voice quality that pierces the listener, who wants to escape as speedily as possible. Sometimes the speaker begins at a normal volume but escalates the intensity as speech continues. Young children, particularly, may talk louder than necessary and appear to be unable to speak at low volume.

Causation. When a student with a loud voice comes to attention, his hearing acuity should be checked since mild losses (especially temporary ones) may cause an unconscious increase in vocal intensity. Sometimes the speaker hears normally but is unable to monitor the volume of his own voice successfully. Some aggressive or insecure personalities who wish to gain and maintain control of verbal interchanges frequently use excessive volume to overpower other speakers. Certain families foster the development of constantly loud speech. Children who are learning to express themselves in large and noisy families may adopt a habitually loud voice as the best way to get a response. People who work around noisy machinery, in crowded workplaces, or where they must be heard across distance often continue to speak with loud volume even in conversational settings. Certain abnormalities in mental functioning seem to cause the disordered speaker to talk loudly, perhaps in an attempt to focus his own attention. Mentally handicapped individuals frequently talk in loud voices, which seems to be an aspect of their limited ability to judge the appropriateness of their behavior.

Implications. Speakers with abnormally loud speech are penalized in social situations because their irritating voices subtract (as well as distract) from the content they wish to communicate. The loud-voiced speaker may be perceived as arrogant and overbearing, although his social behavior is beyond reproach. Professional opportunities as well as personal relationships may be lost because of listener judgments based on voice volume in social situations. Excessive volume may contribute to the formation of nodules or polyps on the vocal folds if there is also tension and trauma over a length of time. Laryngitis often is an immediate symptom and a warning to modify vocal behavior.

CORRECTION Modify these strategies according to the student's learning style, needs, and age.

1. *Softly.* Ask the student to read 10 prepared sentences (easy reading level) at reduced volume. Suggest that he think of a sleeping baby being nearby.
2. *Picture This.* Give the student a picture of people engaged in an interesting activity and ask him to tell a story about it, keeping his voice at a lowered volume. Repeat with pictures until the student has talked for about 10 minutes with normal speech volume.
3. *Relate.* Encourage the student to relate personal experiences or tell about a TV program, incorporating the lowered speech volume into his spontaneous conversation. Listen for any increase in vocal intensity and indicate by moving your hand in a downward direction that he is to lower his speech volume.
4. *Monitor.* Consult with the student's parents and teachers about the problem of loudness. Ask them to monitor the intensity of the student's speech and indicate with the downward hand movement when he should lower his voice.
5. *Secret.* Give the student a passage of easy reading and tell him to maintain his voice volume at a confidential level, as though it were secret material.
6. *Soft Words.* Have the student read this word list, modifying his voice to match the meaning of the words.

soft	baby	feathers
squishy	snowflakes	velvet
slippery	lullaby	clouds

7. *Hearing Check.* Counsel the student concerning the effects of a loud conversational volume on the listeners. Check the hearing level several times at various times of the day to determine if fluctuations in acuity may be maintaining the loud speech volume. Ask if the student has allergies that may flare up intermittently and interfere with the normal ability to monitor one's own speech volume. Recommend that the student have his ear canals cleaned by an otologist to dislodge any impacted cerumen (wax).
8. *TV Homework.* Help the student choose a role model on TV who has a pleasant, well-modulated voice. Realize that since the student must genuinely admire the person, the final choice must be his. Encourage the student to watch the TV personality frequently and attempt to imitate his or her voice pattern. If possible, obtain several minutes of videotape of the person speaking and view it together with the student. Discuss the intensity level of the person's speech and the contribution it makes to the listener's impression.

24. TOO SOFT VOICE

DETECTION This is a problem if a student over 6 years of age displays:

- Unintelligible speech due to weak volume
- Lack of vitality in voice
- Conversational volume that is softer than that of other speakers
- Speech volume that is inappropriate for the situation

Description. Students sometimes speak with very low volume, making their speech so different that it interferes with communication. These speakers may speak with high, low, or normal pitch but seem to have no ability to project their voices. Their words often seem to be produced with little or no effort and minimal regard for the listener. Persons with too soft voices seldom recognize any communication problem resulting from their speech. When they speak, the listener must give close attention, and even then the message may not be completely intelligible. This causes the listener embarrassment and after several unsatisfactory exchanges, the conversation may languish and the speaker with the soft voice will never know why.

Causation. A too soft voice may be the result of a frail physical condition, an indication of an abnormal physiological state of the laryngeal or respiratory mechanism, or a manifestation of a reticent personality. After clearance by a medical examination, the speech pathologist may search out remedial avenues. The weak voice is often seen in combination with other vocal abnormalities, such as breathiness and intermittent aphonia. The soft voice may be psychoneurotic in origin and relate to tension, anxiety, repression, inhibition, insecurity, or fear. Sometimes the speaker has never learned proper breathing for the production of speech or is speaking at an abnormal pitch. The speaker may have chosen the soft speech as representative of gentility or other desirable qualities. Occasionally, a student appears to derive some satisfaction from the extra attention directed to her when her speech is difficult to hear.

Implications. Individuals with soft voices are also frequently penalized in social situations. Their voices are often lost in the crowd, and engaging in one-to-one conversation with them requires more effort than most listeners are willing to exert. The speaker with the soft voice may be viewed as ineffectual or dependent and therefore may be eliminated from consideration for professional opportunities.

CORRECTION Modify these strategies according to the student's learning style, needs, and age.

1. *Dr. First.* A weak voice that reflects poor physical health must be dealt with through medical treatment before voice therapy can be effective.

2. *Stand Straight.* Begin with respiration and the production of a strong airstream. Direct the student to stand with her feet 6–8 inches apart, shoulders back but relaxed, pelvis tucked so "the dining room is upstairs and the sitting room is downstairs," and knees slightly flexed. Now tell the student to imagine that there is a string from the top of her head from which her body is suspended.

3. *Breathe Deeply.* Demonstrate deep breathing and help the student to imitate, placing her hand on her abdomen to illustrate the expansion due to optimal inhalation. Raise your hand as you breathe in with closed mouth, and lower it as you breathe out with open mouth. Instruct the student to practice deep breathing with forceful exhalation, but attempt only 5–6 in sequence because the unaccustomed oxygen intake could cause dizziness.

4. *Say "Ah!"* Direct the student to say "ah" on exhalation, sustaining the tone without breaks in phonation. Encourage the her to gradually increase the volume on successive trials. Tell the student to stop if there is a sensation of strain or discomfort. Repeat the exercise after vocal rest, returning to a softer volume and increase as the effort is tolerated.

5. *Soft Voice.* Direct the student to stand across the room from you and read (easy reading level) a paragraph aloud. Remind the student when volume is too low: "I can't hear you!"

6. *Cheers!* Tell the student that she is to be a cheerleader for the high school team and is to practice the cheers with you. Try this cheer:
   Give me an A. Give me an L.
   Give me an L. —ALL!
   Give me an S. Give me a T.
   Give me an A-T-E!
   ALLSTATE, ALLSTATE, YEAH!

7. *Application.* Instruct the student that she is to demonstrate excitement as she uses an unplugged telephone to:
   - Call the fire department and report a kitchen fire at her home address, emphasizing the need to hurry.
   - Call the police department and report an accident between a car with 3 occupants and a pick-up truck carrying crates of chickens that have fallen and burst open.
   - Call a friend who is busy doing her homework and tell her you made an A on your test, which means you can go to the party after all.
   The teacher or therapist will take the role of listener and ask appropriate questions.

8. *Speak Up.* Explain to the student that it is important that she projects her voice with enough volume to be heard. Ask the student to match the volume of your voice as you slowly read a list of 1-syllable words. You read one word, the student reads the next, and then continue alternating in that manner through the remainder of the list. Next, tape record as you again read the list but in reverse order, together. Place the tape recorder across the room, set the volume at a low level, and ask the student to repeat the words. Determine how many words of each voice are intelligible to her.

CHAPTER 8

QUALITY

25. HOARSE VOICE

DETECTION Notice if students (especially boys of 8–10) display:

- Chronic hoarseness
- Reduced vocal range
- Repeated loss of voice
- Frequent laryngitis
- Some inaudible speech sounds
- Difficulty making oral responses in class

Description. Hoarseness is easily recognized by the low, husky, grating voice. The speaker usually appears to be straining to produce even those defective sounds and may evidence voice breaks when phonation ceases completely. Vocal range is limited and the speech lacks both vitality and variety.

Causation. The laryngologist who examines the speaker will determine the presence or absence of abnormal physiology or pathological conditions of the larynx and associated structures. Among the conditions that might be reported are laryngeal tumors, neural lesions affecting the larynx, paralysis of one or both vocal folds, weakness of the phonatory musculature, chronic infection of the respiratory tract, or irritation from external materials. If none of these or other structural conditions is identified, the speech pathologist may conclude that the hoarseness is functional and, after consultation with the physician, attempt to alleviate the symptoms. The hoarseness may be produced by misuse or abuse of the larynx and pharynx. Nodules sometimes form on the edges of the vocal folds as a result of speaking with too much intensity and perhaps at too low a pitch. Tension produced by vocalists who strain the voice causes abnormal contact of the vocal folds, building up the calluslike nodules. Contact ulcers also may be the result of vocal abuse, usually occurring at a different location on the vocal folds and resulting in husky to hoarse voice quality. Misuse of the voice occurs as a result of a lack of synchrony among the components of the phonological system: breathing, phonation, and resonation. This may be due to pitch, intensity, breath pressure, the channeling of the airstream, or a combination of factors.

Implications. The student with a hoarse voice may dismiss it as "just laryngitis" or "because I yelled at the game last night." Any persistent hoarseness should be referred for medical attention. The student may regard his aberrant voice as distinctive or similar to that of a popular entertainer, indicating the need for counseling as to the long-term effects of chronic hoarseness. The student can be advised to avoid smoking or smoke-filled areas and to be aware of vocal fold tenderness during respiratory infections. Continued misuse or abuse of the voice may make it necessary to recommend a period of complete voice rest, with or without surgery to remove the nodules or ulcers. The student who does not learn to use his voice correctly loses access to a number of professions that require a considerable amount of speaking.

CORRECTION After obtaining medical clearance, modify these strategies according to the student's learning style, needs, and age.

1. *Vocal Counselor.* Counsel the student concerning the benefits of good vocal usage, the hazards of voice misuse, and the indicators of tension and fatigue.
2. *Let Go.* Teach the student the principles of progressive relaxation by contraction and relaxation of sets of muscles from the toes to the scalp while lying flat on a firm surface.
3. *Around and Around.* Demonstrate controlled, easy breathing for speech. Encourage the student to relax the laryngeal area by yawning and by rolling his head in a circular motion.
4. *Exhale.* Instruct the student to take a deep breath and exhale with a sustained "h," produced without a vowel and without forcing. Repeat, reminding the student to control the airstream in an effort to prolong exhalation.
5. *Hah!* Demonstrate how the student is to inhale deeply and then exhale while vocalizing [ha] (hah) in effortless phonation. Repeat using the syllables [hɔ] (haw), [hʌ] (huh), [hi] (he), and [haɪ] (high) in turn. Encourage the student to try for steady phonation, but warn against forcing the sound.
6. *Read Easy.* Prepare a list of words at the appropriate reading level that begin with "h." Ask the student to read them aloud in order to practice the initiation of phonation without hard glottal attack.
7. *Read More.* Prepare lists of words beginning with the letters "wh" and with "y" for the student to read for further practice in easy phonation.
8. *Easy Does It.* Prepare sentences containing words beginning with the letters "h," "wh," and "y." Ask the student to maintain easy phonation while reading aloud sentences such as these:
   He had a whole hamburger.
   His wheels are yellow.
   Herbert said, "yes," he had heard the hounds.
   Whistle while you work and whittle.
   When will white horses walk away?
   Have Heather whisper his name.
9. *TLC.* Suggest that the student take frequent sips of liquids throughout the day and gargle with warm salt water occasionally.

26. NASAL VOICE

DETECTION Watch for the student who exhibits:

- Hypernasality in conversational speech
- Higher than normal pitch

Description. Hypernasal speech calls attention to itself in most regions. There are some areas in which a certain amount of hypernasality is the norm, however. "Country bumpkins" or "hillbillies" are sometimes portrayed as having a nasal twang, as are sophisticated big-city types. The pitch is ordinarily raised above the optimum level when an excessive amount of nasopharyngeal resonance is present. Hypernasal speech is seldom regarded as normal and most listeners find it at least mildly unpleasant. Occasionally, a speaker produces hyponasal (denasal) speech. This may be due to a temporary or chronic nasal congestion that occludes the air passageway. That speaker might say something similar to "How benny tibes bust I tell you?" Sometimes students have extremely large adenoids which partially close off the nasal passage; medical intervention is often advised.

Causation. Excessive nasality (hypernasality) occurs primarily during vowel production and is produced as the airstream is allowed to flow through the nasal passage inappropriately. This occurs when there is only partial closure of the nasal port and results in inharmonic vibration. It is, therefore, a resonance problem that can be caused by the physical structure of the oronasopharyngeal cavities or by undue tension of the muscles and tissues of the laryngopharyngeal area. The effectiveness of the velopharyngeal seal is important, and insufficiency in this area may result from various causes. A laryngologist can examine the structure and functioning of the soft palate (velum) to determine if surgery could improve the action of the mechanism as it elevates to effect closure. A tonsillectomy or adenoidectomy can damage the tissue of the velum or its controlling musculature. The removal of the tonsils and/or adenoids may be enough to cause hypernasality until the speaker can learn to adjust to the loss of the tissue mass which may have contributed to complete closure of the nasal port.

Implications. The student who exhibits hypernasality does not ordinarily experience academic problems as a result of her speech pattern. There may very well be difficulties in social interaction with peers if the speech is viewed as markedly different. Often a student with hypernasal speech is reluctant to recite in class or carry out assignments that require speaking before a group. Chances of success in certain careers, such as teaching, acting, or holding political office, may be diminished by a hypernasal speech pattern.

CORRECTION After obtaining medical clearance, modify these strategies according to the student's learning style, needs, and age.

1. *Hear It.* The first step in remediating hypernasality is auditory training. The speaker must learn to distinguish the difference between a nasal sound and a not nasal sound. Pronounce this list of words, some with and some without hypernasality, and ask the listener to name them nasal or nonnasal:

nine	telephone	ransom
feet	Harry	blanket
banana	think	blame

2. *Feel It.* To help students learn the concept of nasality, have them place their forefingers along the side of the bony parts of their noses. Have them produce [m], [n], and [ŋ] (ng) while they feel the nasal vibrations. Have them repeat words with these nasal sounds:

mama	ring	name
no	sang	number
moon	bringing	length
none	morning	string

3. *Blow Out.* Retraining of the vocal mechanism may require stimulation of stronger velar action, which is the object of this exercise. Demonstrate for the student how to blow out the cheeks and explode the air forcefully, then easily, through puckered lips.

4. *Balloon.* Give the student a soft balloon to blow up; when it is filled with air, direct the student to allow the air to flow back into her mouth slowly until her cheeks are distended.

5. *Puh-Tuh-Kuh.* Direct the student to prepare to produce the [p] and hold for a few seconds while sensing the firm closure of the nasal port before exploding it in conjunction with the sounds [a] (ah) and [ɔ] (aw); repeat the exercise using the plosives [t] and [k].

6. *Hold It.* Direct the student to read these sentences and prolong the implosive phase of each stop consonant. Demonstrate for young children.
    A big dog grabbed a bite of biscuit.
    Bo-Bo, the goat, butts the pigs, ducks, and geese.
    The big, bad wolf said, "I'll huff and I'll puff and blow your house down."
    Betty said, "Don't put bitter butter on my bread."

7. *Through a Straw.* The development of oral pressure can be helped by blowing exercises, such as these:
    • Blow through a plastic straw to move feathers, confetti, or tissue pieces all to one side of a dividing line in a shallow box without blowing them out of the box.
    • Blow ping-pong balls across a table or up an inclined plane, increasing the angle as strength increases.

8. *Relax.* Emphasize a pattern of production that utilizes a relaxed jaw, a large mouth opening, and mobile tongue tip and lips. Have the student stand before the mirror, yawn, and then produce [ɛ] (eh), [a] (ah), [ʌ] (uh), [ɔ] (aw), [o] (oh), maintaining a relaxed jaw with open mouth and laryngeal area.

27. BREATHY VOICE

DETECTION Notice the student who:

- Exhibits excessive breathiness when speaking
- Produces weak speech volume
- Inhales frequently

Description. Excessive breathiness in the voice is not unpleasant for the listener, but it does distract from the speaker's message. In addition, the breathy voice is usually soft in volume due to the inefficient use of the airstream. The student who exhibits breathiness frequently must interrupt his comments to inhale again since his air is exhausted, resulting in a broken speech pattern.

Causation. For ideal phonation, the edges of the vocal folds come together throughout their length and are in close enough approximation that air does not escape except when noticeable pressure is exerted. Obviously, irregularities on the edges of the vocal folds will prevent good closure, allowing air to leak out even when the folds are in the closed, vibrating phase. These irregularities may be congenital and simply variants from normal structure. The irregularities may be scars from damage to the vocal folds from swallowing a solid object or from intubation during an operation. Misuse of the voice can cause nodules or even contact ulcers to form on the edges of the vocal folds. In other cases, they could be pathological (tubercular, syphilitic, or cancerous), which is a compelling reason to refer all voice cases for medical examination. The vocal folds may fail to meet because of paralysis of one or both due to traumatization of the controlling vagus nerve through surgery, accident, or disease. The breathiness of laryngitis results from fixation of the arytenoid cartilages due to the mass of tissue preventing the approximation of the vocal folds. Failure of the folds to meet adequately allows the escape of the airstream, producing breathiness. Continued attempts to vocalize can traumatize the swollen tissue and cause further damage, which may have long-lasting effects.

Some women may adopt a breathy voice in an attempt to sound mysterious or sensual. It appears to be completely a matter of choice, since they may revert to a normal voice production when it suits them. Certain famous actresses have made a breathy voice symbolic of sexual attractiveness.

Implications. A student who has a breathy voice may have difficulty being heard in even a moderately noisy situation. Voice projection is poor so that most conversations must be held at close range. Listeners who pay close attention to a speaker with a breathy voice may still miss some of the message. Classroom recitation may be a burden for both the speaker and listeners, which could have ramifications for social as well as academic achievement.

CORRECTION After obtaining medical clearance, modify these strategies according to the student's learning style, needs, and age.

1. *No Abuse.* A breathy voice may be a concomitant of hoarseness; therefore, remediation of the vocal misuse, if that was the precipitating factor, will diminish the breathy quality.
2. *Counsel.* When breathiness is due to chronic laryngitis, the student should be counseled concerning preventative measures; awareness of sensations of tension, fatigue, and pain; and the danger of permanent vocal damage.
3. *Diagram.* Prepare a diagram to illustrate the vocal anatomy and discuss the process of phonation with the student. For example, you might say, "Air is drawn into the lungs, then pushed up and out through the larynx (seen as the Adam's apple). When the vocal folds (or cords) in the larynx are closed, the escaping air opens them and causes them to vibrate, producing sound. As the sound moves through the mouth and nose, it is changed by movement of the palate, lips, and tongue." While you describe the process to students, point out each step on the diagram. Vary the complexity of the explanation according to student ability and need, but in each case, emphasize the need to expel the air in a slow, steady stream for best speech production.
4. *AH-H.* Help the student learn to control breath expulsion. Direct him to take a deep abdominal breath, clasp his hands over his diaphragm, and try for a steady relaxation as he intones "a" for as long as possible. Try this exercise at the beginning, middle, and end of every session, using a stopwatch to time each phonation; chart improvements to illustrate progress.
5. *Count.* Instruct the student to inhale deeply, and then exhale slowly while counting from 1 to 10 as the leader indicates the beat by touching a pencil to the table (to prevent hurried counting).
6. *Hum Along.* Encourage the student to hum the tunes to favorite songs while others in the group guess the titles.
7. *Self-Critique.* Tape record the student reading an easy passage, play it back, and note the words he says with breathiness and without. Tape again, reminding the student to control the breathiness as much as possible. Play the second recording for the student to analyze for progress.
8. *Announcer.* Advise the student that he is to practice being a TV news announcer and the presenter of a sales message for a commercial. Prepare passages to be read as local news and a sales pitch for pizza. Emphasize the need for clear speech, breath control, and a firm, rapid delivery. Tape record the student's presentations and play back for discussion concerning speech quality.

REFLECTIONS

1. In Part III, voice disorders involving pitch, intensity, and quality were described, accompanied by reminders that referral should be made for medical examination before instituting any corrective measures. Explain the reasons for such a recommendation and list possible developments if the medical examination were not obtained.

2. An individual's voice often provides insight concerning self-image. Think of speakers you know whose voice pitch is unusually high or unusually low. Do their voices complement their personalities? How would you approach changing voice pitch with those individuals? Write the first 3 steps of your proposed management.

3. In Chapter 6, monotone pitch is described as distracting from the speaker's communicative competence. Review the CORRECTION strategies for a monotone voice and then choose one to demonstrate with a peer.

4. As you observe in elementary classrooms, you will have an opportunity to hear most of the children in the class speak. Note the percentage who speak too loudly or too softly in a specific classroom. Later, observe those same children on the playground and compare their in-class and out-of-class voices. Is this important in planning correction strategies?

5. Chapter 7 contains a description of a hoarse voice, followed by a discussion of causative factors. Compile a list of avoidable situations or behaviors that may contribute to the development of a hoarse voice.

6. Hypernasality is a voice characteristic common in some regions or among certain groups. Reread Skill 26 and complete Activity 2. Repeat the words in Activity 1, saying them first with excess nasality, and then correcting the production by redirecting the airstream appropriately. Check for good sounds by feeling the vibrations along the nasal bone.

7. Prepare a diagram of the vocal anatomy, as suggested in Activity 3 of Skill 27. Practice giving an oral explanation of the process of phonation that would be suitable for a fifth-grade class. Experiment with ways to illustrate the action of the air setting the vocal folds in vibration.

8. It is difficult to be aware of the pitch, intensity, and quality of our own voices because those aspects are altered as the bones of the head aid in conducting sounds to the inner ear. Tape record your voice as you read a short passage and as you engage in spontaneous conversation with another person. As you listen to your recorded voice, listen for disturbances of pitch, intensity, or quality. Compare your recorded voice with that of a peer.

9. Voice quality is sometimes affected by certain physical changes on the edges of the vocal folds. Refer to the causation section of Skill 25, Hoarse Voice, and be able to describe the problems and how they affect voice production.

10. The reader is urged to seek further information; the following books discuss some of the topics included in this chapter. Compare and contrast the information presented and the remediation techniques suggested.

Andrews, M., & Summers, A. (1987). *Voice therapy for adolescents.* San Diego, CA: College-Hill Press.

Baer, T., Sasaki, C., & Harris, K. S. (1987). *Laryngeal function in phonation and respiration.* San Diego, CA: College-Hill Press.

Brodnitz, F. (1983). *Keep your voice healthy* (2nd ed.). San Diego, CA: College-Hill Press.

Duran, E. (1988). *Teaching the moderately and severely handicapped student and autistic adolescent: With particular attention to bilingual special education.* Springfield, IL: Charles C. Thomas.

Hirano, M., Kirchner, J. A., & Bless, D. (1987). *Neurolaryngology: Recent advances.* San Diego, CA: College-Hill Press.

Johns-Lewis, C. (1986). *Intonation in discourse.* San Diego, CA: College-Hill Press.

Johnson, T. S. (1985). *Vocal abuse reduction program.* San Diego, CA: College-Hill Press.

Katz, R., Davidoff, M., & Wolfe, G. (1988). *Improving communication in Parkinson's disease: A guide for patient, family, and friends.* Danville, IL: Interstate.

Leith, W. R. & Johnston, R. G. (1986). *Handbook of voice therapy for the school clinician.* San Diego, CA: College-Hill Press.

Oyer, H. J. (1987). *Speech, language, and hearing disorders: A guide for the teacher.* San Diego, CA: College-Hill Press.

Shames, G. H., & Wiig, E. H. (Eds.) (1990). *Human communication disorders: An introduction* (3rd ed.). Columbus, OH: Charles E. Merrill.

Sies, L. (1987). *Voice and voice disorders: A handbook for clinicians.* Springfield, IL: Charles C. Thomas.

Stemple, J. C. & Holcomb, B. J. (1988). *Effective voice and articulation.* Columbus, OH: Charles E. Merrill.

Wilson, D. K. (1987). *Voice problems of children* (3rd ed.). Baltimore, MD: Williams and Wilkins.

PART IV

FLUENCY

Dysfluency is a disorder that can affect members of any society and speakers of any language. There are specific references to stuttering in the Bible, by Aristotle of Greece, in medieval and old Anglo-Saxon records, and right down to the 20th century. The universality of dysfluency is demonstrated by researchers who have found terms for stuttering in almost every culture and language investigated. Attempts have been made to determine the number of dysfluent speakers in the general population. Since the behavior is variable over time, both prevalence (percentage of stutterers in a given population at a certain time) and incidence (percentage of persons classified as stutterers at some time in their lives) estimates should be considered. Prevalence has been estimated at .1/2% to 1% of 12-year-old students and incidence at 3% (persons who stuttered for 6 months or more).

There are many definitions of dysfluency, because dysfluency is a many-faceted disorder. Some authorities describe it as an emotional or psychological problem; some believe that it results from neurological dysfunction. Others see it as the result of illness or of environmental influences, while some describe it in terms of the feelings of the speaker. For the purposes of this discussion, it is helpful to list certain behaviors generally agreed to constitute stuttering.

Stuttering is an interruption in the fluency of speech caused by dysrhythmic silences and interjections, struggle to produce sounds, repetitions of speech sounds, or prolongation of single sounds that occur frequently and involuntarily. This behavior interferes with communication and may be accompanied by facial grimaces, irrelevant body movements, and other evidence of tension in the speaker.

In Chapter 9, the most common behavior identified as stuttering, repetition, is described according to variations in production, tempo, and position of occurrence within an utterance. A differentiation is made between normal and abnormal repetitions and between beginning and later stutterers. Prolongations, another component of stuttering speech, may be an attempt by the speaker to avoid repeating beginning sounds, but the result is to add another abnormal behavior to the speech pattern. Descriptions of the physical action are followed by mention of psychological factors that may be involved.

The most devastating aspect of stuttering may be the occurrence of a phonatory block when the speaker simply cannot produce the desired sound. The block is painful for both listener and speaker, as the stutterer strains and struggles to say the word that refuses to leave his or her mouth. This is a serious speech problem that often requires intensive and extensive therapy. Chapter 9 concludes with some of the associated behaviors adopted by secondary or confirmed stutterers. In their desperate attempts to initiate and maintain smooth speech, some students unconsciously incorporate certain physical movements that may have contributed to speech improvement at one time but are no longer productive.

Other dysfluencies are discussed in Chapter 10. Cluttering is a fluency disorder characterized by an excessive rate of speech, poor articulation, omission and repetition of words and phrases, and disorganized sentence structure. Particular attention is given to the ways in which cluttering differs from stuttering. It should be remembered that dysfluent speech may be situational and can encompass one, some, or all of the behaviors described in Chapters 9 and 10.

Family members, friends, teachers, and speech pathologists should be aware of the psychological effects of stuttering speech. The speaker often develops feelings of fear, anxiety, anger, guilt, and self-disgust, which may be expressed or repressed. It is not easy for others to be closely associated with a person who stutters, for the feelings generated by the stutter's abnormal speech spill over into every part of his or her life. Other types of dysfluencies may not carry these negative feelings for the speaker, although they may be equally distressing to the listener. The primary consideration when attempting to remediate dysfluent speech should be to continue to confirm the value of the individual. The object of therapy may be to help the person be as fluent as possible and to develop a healthy attitude of self-acceptance.

CHAPTER 9 /
STUTTERING

28. REPETITIONS

DETECTION Watch for the student who:

- Repeats two- or three-word phrases
- Repeats words
- Repeats singular sounds or parts of words

Description. Repetitions are probably the most commonly identifiable form of stuttering behavior. They seem to appear quite often at the beginnings of syntactic units—more specifically, at the beginnings of sentences, clauses, verb phrases, noun phrases, or prepositional phrases. Stutterers will repeat two- and three-word phrases, but usually the repetitions involve words, syllables, and single sounds (e.g., She-she-she t-t-t-t-took my ba-ba-ba-baseball). It must be noted that repetitions are sometimes exhibited by normal speakers, but they tend to repeat phrases and whole words, not syllables or sounds. The few syllabic repetitions that a normal speaker may show occur at the same tempo as the rest of their syllables. Stutterers repeat syllables in a jerky manner. The repetitions seem to be arrested or terminated suddenly by interruption of the breath stream. Syllabic repetitions vary in rate among different stutterers and in a single individual stutterer at different times. In beginning stutterers, repetitions tend to occur with the same timing of delivery as their fluent speech. However, as the disorder progresses, the rate of delivery of repetitions becomes much faster. Sometimes the rate of syllabic repetitions is faster than the stutterer can actually produce voluntarily.

Causation. Repetitions may result from the stutterer being unable to organize the completion of her utterance. She experiences a syntactic breakdown of sorts and uses a repetition to maintain verbal momentum. Repetitions could also be an anticipatory coping mechanism used by the stutterer to stave off or postpone a perceived breakdown. Some experts postulate the repetitions are triggered by some sort of sensors in a feedback loop. When these sensors detect an error in speech, recycling in the form of repetitions occurs. The error is either in the articulation of a sound or the timing of accompanying respiration or phonation.

Implications. It is important to distinguish between normal dysfluency and stuttering. One means of differentiation is to clearly define the type of repetition that the speaker is exhibiting. Smaller units of repetition imply more severe stuttering. Determine the frequency of occurrence for repetitions (percent of dysfluency per 100, 200, etc. words). When frequency exceeds 5%, the speech can be considered abnormally dysfluent.

CORRECTION Modify these strategies for the student's learning style, needs, and age.

1. *Fluency Rule.* Establish the rule that the student should say a word only once. Explain to the student that to be understood, she does not have to repeat words. Have her take note of your speech and the speech of friends and other adults to determine if sounds or words are spoken more than once. Have her compare these observations to records of her own speech.

2. *Reducing Occurrence.* Use a tape recorder to sample the student's spontaneous speech at the beginning or end of each therapy session. Assist the student with identifying her repetitions and work toward having her do this independently. Develop a chart to graph the data. Target specific levels of reduction for reward. Regularly repeat the activity and review with the student her progress.

3. *Cancellation.* Instruct the student to stop speaking when she experiences a repetition. She should pause, think about what she wants to say, take a breath, and say it. Have her hold on to the first sound and move gently into the rest of the word, and then the rest of the utterance.

4. *Response Patterns.* Develop response patterns that are reflective of conversation that might occur during the student's school day and at home. Vary the structure of the interchanges so that the student is involved in initiation and response. Sample patterns might include these:
    - Where is your homework?
      It's in my notebook.
    - What's our assignment?
      It's written on the board.
    - Why are you tardy?
      The bus was late.
    - Where is our bus?
      It's over there.

   Encourage the student to expand response patterns spontaneously. This will allow her to build confidence for spontaneity in a controlled situation.

5. *Facing Fears.* Have the student describe how she feels when she stutters. If this is difficult for her, provide a list of possibilities from which to choose. Use this activity to initiate discussion. It is important that the student identify and face her feelings if she is to overcome them.

6. *Generalization. In Class.* Ask another professional who works with the student to collect random data samples of the student's repetitions and provide you with this information. Have that person encourage the student to answer questions, at least 1 each day, even if the response is just a single word. *At Home.* Have the student read a recipe and then restate the directions for someone who is cooking. Make sure that family members are aware of her fluency rule so they can help monitor her speech. *Community Experience.* Have the student place an order at a fast-food restaurant. Prepare for this situation by roleplaying with possible response patterns. After each simulation or the experience itself, have her describe the experience and her overall communicative behaviors, both fluent and dysfluent.

29. PROLONGATIONS

DETECTION Watch for the student who:
- Lengthens vowels and continues consonants, particularly at the beginnings of words
- Fixates the position of the articulators for the production of plosive consonants

Description. Prolongations are demonstrated by all confirmed stutterers. Normal speakers hold on to sounds only briefly. Stutterers show a longer duration. Because normal speaking is characterized by continuous movement, even slight prolongations of posture or sound are conspicuous. The stutterer may hold on to the [m] for a longer than normal time when saying the word "mother" or may position the tongue and jaw to form the [t] in "tea" and hold the position too long. Sometimes this type of prolongation will be preceded by silent rehearsal movements of the articulators. When the stutterer is prolonging a sound, it is not always smooth. There may be fluctuations in volume, airflow, pitch, and tension. Although prolongations may coexist with repetitions in a stutterer's dysfluency pattern, they do seem to develop later than repetitions and increase as the disorder progresses.

Causation. Many different possibilities may explain the presence of prolongations in dysfluent speech. Because they are found to coexist with repetitions, they may result from the stutterer's attempt to prevent a repetition by extending the particular sound that is likely to be repeated. The stutterer may also be afraid of stopping his airflow or voice, so he uses prolongation as a time-gaining device to get ready for the remainder of the utterance. Some stutterers may use prolongations to avoid a stuttering block by keeping the vocal folds vibrating. This allows them to proceed without a laryngospasm. Many experts believe that prolongations are indicators of the fear that causes approach/avoidance. The stutterer's intent and desire for verbal communication are temporarily overcome by the fear of stuttering. Sounds are prolonged as the stutterer attempts to get past the conflict. There may be no satisfactory explanation for an individual stutterer; however, the end result is a problem that can be described in terms of rhythm and timing.

Implications. Because prolongations are characteristic of established stuttering behavior, the therapeutic program will likely address prolongations in addition to other stuttering behavior. Although a difficult task, it may be helpful to try to target the reason the stutterer is prolonging sounds; this may help with selecting the therapeutic strategy for eliminating this behavior. For example, if the stutterer prolongs only selected sounds, it will only be necessary to target these sounds. If he prolongs every time he anticipates a block, alternative strategies for preventing blocks will need to be taught. It will also be very helpful for the student to become aware of the actual length of his prolongations. Many stutterers unrealistically estimate the duration of their prolongations. To some, what seems to be only a brief duration may actually be an extended time, while others find momentary prolongations painfully lengthy.

CORRECTION Modify these strategies for the student's learning style, needs, and age.

1. *Awareness.* Provide the student with a list of sounds. Have him check the ones he feels may cause him to prolong. Compare this information with data you collect from spontaneous speech samples. Analyze and discuss the findings with the student.

2. *Fluency Rule.* Establish the rule that the student must not prolong sounds when he speaks. Explain that fluent speech is made up of concise sounds that flow together to form words and sentences. With young children, try using long and short pieces of rough material to illustrate the rule. Have the student repeat prolonged sounds or words as he rules his finger over the long piece of material. Have him rub his finger over the short piece of material as he repeats short sounds and words. A stopwatch is a helpful tool for older students. Have each student time his speech production, beginning with single-syllable words. Allow no more than 2 seconds per word or syllable. As the student becomes more adept with using the stopwatch, expand the exercise so that he times his production of phrases and sentences.

3. *Voluntary Stuttering.* This activity encourages the student to consciously imitate his own dysfluency. The voluntary prolongations should be characterized by the easy onset of the first sound or syllable of a word or by gently prolonging the entire word. Encourage the student to use this style of talking as a replacement for his usual stuttering behavior. The premise here is that this intentional stuttering will reduce fear by having the stutterer voluntarily do what he is most afraid of. Awareness of the mechanics may also help to increase metacognitive behaviors as well as to eliminate overavoidance behaviors.

4. *Reducing Occurrence.* Using a tape recorder, obtain a spontaneous speech sample at the beginning of each therapy session. Obtain a baseline on the frequency and duration of the prolongations. Teach the student to count and time his prolongations. Establish levels of reduction for reward, chart the data to provide a visual representation of progress, and regularly analyze and discuss the results with the student, involving him in planning further therapy.

5. *Targeting.* To determine if prolongations are word or sound related, select an oral reading passage and have the student read it to you. Make a note of the sounds or words that are prolonged. Then ask him to summarize the passage orally and compare the 2 samples. Have him complete these same activities with his parents and a friend. Compare the results of each sample to determine if a trend is established.

6. *Generalization. In Class.* Have the student make the morning announcements, practicing his current fluency rule. *At Home.* Have the student time the syllable production of one of his favorite television characters to practice analysis of fluent speech. *Community Experience.* Have the student practice his fluency rule each time he speaks with a favorite neighbor and then report and critique the experience.

30. HESITATIONS

DETECTION Watch for the student who:
- • Pauses before phrases, words, or sounds within words
- • Uses filler syllables between words or phrases
- • Uses stereotyped expressions at the beginning of an utterance or between words and phrases

Description. Hesitations as stuttering behavior are characterized by pauses in speaking, the use of filler syllables, and stereotyped expression. This behavior is generally found in stutterers who are also exhibiting full-blown stuttering block accompanied by signs of physical struggle. Filler syllables and stereotyped expressions may also be defined as interjections. "Um," "er," "ah," and "uh" are all common interjections used by the stutterer to fill pauses. Expressions such as "well," "let me see," and "you know" are stereotypical utterances that stutterers also interject when hesitating.

Causation. Pauses may be the result of the stutterer's awareness of her fluency problem. The student may be extremely sensitive to sounds or words that she feels cause her to stutter. In an effort to keep from stuttering, she stops speaking before the particular word or sounds occurs. The use of filler syllables and stereotyped expressions may also be interpreted as a postponement tactic used to avoid stuttering. The interjections fill what would otherwise be a silent interval. This may occur because the stutterer knows that filled pauses are probably perceived by the listener as being shorter in duration than empty pauses. In normal speech, hesitations most often indicate that the speaker is searching for a word or form of expression. She is able to maintain verbal momentum and prevent silent gaps. For the stutterer, hesitations allow her to bypass possible spasmodic breakdown and then regain some sense of self-control as she waits for the fear to ebb. Hesitations have also been identified as a means for the stutterer to compel the listener into completing an utterance when she has lost control.

Implications. In that hesitations are generally exhibited in addition to other forms of stuttering behavior, the therapeutic program will need to address the hesitations in conjunction with the other behaviors. It will be necessary to determine the frequency of occurrence as well as the duration of the hesitations because such pauses and interjections also are commonly exhibited by fluent speakers but to a lesser degree. Duration and frequency can be identified best by recording spontaneous speech samples and then counting the number of hesitations that are present per each 100, 200, or 500 words. Identify the type or types of hesitations that are occurring. If the stutterer is simply pausing or ceasing to speak, then the duration of each pause can be timed. If the stutterer is hesitating by employing filler syllables of stereotyped expressions, the duration should be determined by counting the number of times a particular expression is used for each instance of stuttering. It should be noted that stutterers will sometimes combine several expressions into one hesitation (e.g., I uh, um, well, you know, I was there yesterday).

CORRECTION Modify these strategies for the student's learning style, needs, and age.

1. *Awareness.* Prepare several written examples of stuttering hesitations. Have the student read them aloud. See if she can identify her type of stuttering. If the student is young and not reading yet, prepare several tape-recorded examples.

2. *Proper Breathing.* Explain, demonstrate, and guide the student to practice proper (i.e., diaphramatic) breathing for speech production. To highlight both concept and mechanics, demonstrate improper (i.e., clavicular or thoracic) breathing as well. A good exercise for developing appropriate breathing habits is to have the student lie on her back, placing a small book over her diaphragm. The book should rise upon inhalation and fall upon exhalation. Gradually build up to the point at which the student can comfortably practice for 10 minutes per session. After the technique is established, have the student read aloud or speak as she does this.

3. *Fluency Rule.* Instruct the student to use a slow, steady rate of speech production. The intent here is to allow the student time to think ahead, organize her thoughts, and mentally prepare for each word. For young children, using symbolic therapy materials, such as turtles and snails, may be helpful. By stressing even, deliberate speech, the student may eliminate her need for hesitation.

4. *Reducing Occurrence.* After identifying the types of hesitations that the student exhibits, begin working toward eliminating them one by one. For example, if the student is in the habit of using "uh" as a filler, establish baseline data on the frequency and duration. Record a spontaneous speech sample during each therapy session. Have the student assist you with counting and determining the duration of the targeted hesitation. Develop a chart to record the data, target specific levels for reward, and regularly discuss and critique progress with the student.

5. *Changing the Behavior.* Select an interjection that the student will be allowed to use during the therapy session. Select a different interjection each session and make the rule that the student must repeat it 5 times each time she uses it. By increasing the student's awareness of her behavior, she may be assisted as well as motivated to gain control over her use of these stereotyped utterances.

6. *Generalization. In Class.* Have the student practice her fluency rule by reading a short paragraph aloud to the class. Or ask the student to participate in choral reading. As fluency improves, also ask her to restate what she has read. *At Home.* Give the student a brief written summary of each therapy session. Ask her first to read it aloud to 1 family member and then try relating the same information to another family member without reading. As she does this, she should practice her fluency rule. *Community Experience.* Have the student participate in any seasonal type of community programs that involve choral reading (e.g., dramatic productions or religious programs) or choral singing (e.g., various types of choirs). This will give the student the opportunity to have a successful speaking experience in a group setting.

31. STUTTERING BLOCKS

DETECTION Watch for the student who:
- Abruptly halts the flow of speech and shows signs of struggle
- Is unable to initiate an utterance and shows signs of struggle

Description. Stuttering blocks are abrupt interruptions in the flow of speech. For a time, the stutterer is literally unable to move or control the speech articulators to produce the intended word. The block occurs in conjunction with the repetitions, prolongations, or hesitations that define the speaker's dysfluency pattern. Characteristics of stuttering blocks are widely varied. Muscles used for speech may become temporarily frozen, blocking the articulation of any phoneme. The stutterer may use starter noises to resume the flow of air for speech production. Visible signs of struggle will be evident as the stutterer attempts to break the block.

Causation. Many stutterers describe a feeling of apprehension before they experience a stuttering block. This is known as the phenomenon of anticipation or expectancy. This aspect of the disorder may interfere the most with communication. Stuttering blocks may arise from fear associated with the stutterer having to speak in certain situations. The fear associated with certain words or speech sounds may also cause the speaker to experience stuttering blocks. The stutterer's anticipation of the block itself may serve as a trigger; however, some stuttering blocks seem to occur without the stutterer having any prior awareness of the onset.

Implications. The stutterer who is blocking often experiences the feeling of having his speech physically halted. This inability to maintain physical control is baffling and disturbing for him. Additionally, feelings of strain and tension become associated with the stuttering block. Several popular therapeutic methods are targeted specifically at stuttering blocks. One approach centers around respiration based upon the assumption that faulty breathing is the culprit responsible for triggering the spasmodic behavior of the vocal folds and prevents the outward flow of air necessary for speech production. Another approach focuses on block corrections, which are designed to help the stutterer solve blocking problems by changing the embedded compulsive responses to more appropriate ones. The corrective strategies described herein embrace both of these approaches. However, regardless of the approach used, the student must feel at ease with the therapy activities in order to be successful in correcting his blocking behavior. To achieve a facilitative comfort level, the therapist and the student should work together to identify and analyze the student's stuttering blocks. Once the student can describe and understand his blocking behavior, he will be better prepared to begin to monitor his speech production and to select and even help design therapeutic activities. Involving the student in planning and implementing therapy will also foster a sense of self-direction and control that will assist with generalization outside of therapy. The use of a third party to monitor performance and progress is often an effective means of encouraging, reinforcing, and maintaining the fluent behavior.

CORRECTION Modify these strategies for the student's learning style, needs, and age.

1. *Awareness.* Provide the student with a list of possible stress situations. Have him identify the ones in which he feels that he is likely to stutter. After the student has identified the situations, target 1 on which to work. Begin by identifying exactly what the situational stressors are (e.g., not having enough time to respond, the possibility of saying the wrong thing, or the chance that he might not be able to stop stuttering). Discuss each stressor. Help the student prepare for the situation by roleplaying.

2. *Easy Onset Speech Production.* Explain, demonstrate, and then guide the student to practice easy onset speech production. After inhalation, exhalation should begin slowly before beginning to speak. Have the student move gently into the first sound of the utterance, making sure that he continues to exhale as he speaks. Stopping the airstream may be what triggers a stuttering block. Have the student practice talking slowly and easily without forcing. Explain that it is all right to stutter, just so it is done easily. The idea is to guide the student to use normal, quiet breathing and become accustomed to not forcing his way out of a block.

3. *Postblock Correction/Cancellation.* Instruct the student to use these steps for postblock correction:
   • First finish saying the word on which the block occurred.
   • Pause.
   • Take a deep breath and relax as the air is exhaled.
   • As you pause and relax, determine if any corrections need to be made.
   • Use easy onset and start speaking again.
   Verbalize each step whenever you note the need for its use.

4. *Preblock Correction.* Instruct the student to use these steps whenever he anticipates blocking:
   • Pause to relax any tension.
   • Visualize abnormal blocking behavior.
   • Determine how to modify the block.
   • Use the easy onset technique to resume speaking.
   Provide a written copy of these steps to students who can easily read them.

5. *Inblock Correction/Pull Out.* Instruct the student to use the following steps if he finds himself in the middle of a block:
   • Deliberately slow down the stuttering by repeating or prolonging.
   • Hold the stuttering long enough to regain control.
   • Discontinue the stuttering by using the easy onset.
   Whenever you note the need for the student to use this strategy, verbalize each step or prompt him with key cues such as "Slow; hold for control; easy."

6. *Generalization. In Class.* Have the student lead the "Pledge of Allegiance" using the easy onset technique. *At Home.* Have the student answer the telephone to practice his block correction strategies. *Community Experience.* Have the student ask for reference information at the public library and practice block correction techniques.

32. ASSOCIATED SYMPTOMS

DETECTION Watch for the student who:

- Displays disordered breathing
- Exhibits unusual eye movement
- Evidences muscular tension
- Produces abnormal vocalizations

Description. There is more to stuttering than the disruption of an individual's speech flow. There are many concomitant features, and they are extremely varied. The description of stuttering must include other visible and audible characteristics, which are often referred to as secondary stuttering characteristics. The associated symptoms listed above should certainly not be considered exhaustive because it is difficult to catalog all of the behaviors developed by each individual stutterer. Disordered breathing may be manifested as clavicular or thoracic breathing, irregular respiratory cycles with prolonged inhalation or exhalation, attempts to speak while inhaling, or complete cessation of breathing. Unusual eye movement is characterized by blinking, fixating, movement from side to side, and rolling the eyes upward. Common muscular tensions include facial grimacing, hand tremors, and jerking of the head, arms, and legs. Changes in vocal quality, odd inflections or sharp shifts in pitch, and severe sounds produced by suddenly stopping and releasing breath with the vocal bands characterize the possible associated vocal abnormalities. Pallor, flushing, or perspiration may be visible as accompanying skin reactions with severe stuttering.

Causation. Experts continue to postulate as to the cause (or causes) of these associated behaviors. They appear to manifest initially to reduce the tension and stress caused by stuttering and seem to be performed automatically and unconsciously when they have persisted for some time. For example, swallowing may indeed give the stutterer some sense of relief, so it becomes embedded in the stuttering act. However, as time goes by and the dysfluency continues, the stutterer must move on to another means to relieve the stress of the block, so he begins coughing. After a while, the coughing becomes ineffective and another associated symptom appears. From this scenario, it is easy to see how severe stuttering evolves to be accompanied by several associated symptoms.

Implications. Some stutterers seem to exhibit few of these symptoms, while others may display a great many. The stutterer is often very aware of her behavior and it is very stressful for her. The therapist should realize that the therapy program for a stutterer with associated symptoms must take on the added dimension of extinguishing these behaviors, as they are often more unacceptable to the listener than the actual stuttering. It is important to analyze and clearly define the associated symptoms with the stutterer. It may be helpful to determine whether the behaviors occur in any particular sequence or are more likely to occur in particular situations. This type of baseline data will be especially useful in designing and implementing corrective strategies.

Periodic analyses of defined symptoms, sequence, and situations across time and treatment also provide direction for refining strategies.

CORRECTION Modify these strategies for the student's learning style, needs, and age.

1. *Awareness.* Provide the student with a checklist of associated behaviors. Have her indicate the ones that she knows she uses to break a stuttering block. Ask her to have a family member, another stutterer, a friend, or another teacher complete the checklist, too. Analyze and discuss the findings with the student. You may find that she was not fully aware of all of her associated behaviors.

2. *Self-Monitoring.* Working with a mirror is one good way to have the student observe what she looks like when she stutters. Seat the student beside you at a mirror. Next, while monitoring her appearance and movements in the mirror, have her read aloud and then retell the reading content or tell you about the most recent episode of her favorite television show. Analyze with the student the appearance of her stuttering behaviors. If possible, periodically videotape the student during similar activities, and then guide the student to review and analyze the tape and perhaps even compare tapes across time to evaluate progress

3. *Fluency Rule.* Establish the rule that the student must use only the necessary muscles and body parts (lips, tongue, jaws, etc.) to talk. Explain and then demonstrate to the student that fluent speech is produced by using the appropriate articulators and that it is not necessary or even helpful to move other muscles or body parts when talking.

4. *Massed Practice.* This technique calls for associated behaviors to be practiced purposely, in a concentrated manner, outside of the stuttering situation. The premise is that bringing these behaviors under conscious control will make them easier to manage. If the stutterer has the habit of blinking her eyes, have her do it purposely, just as she does when she stutters, except while not talking. Have the student vary the timing and speed of the blink.

5. *Changing the Behaviors.* If the student exhibits associated stuttering behaviors in an established pattern, set up a program of change. Take all the behaviors that make up the pattern and rearrange them. Add to or drop behaviors from the pattern. If the student blinks, coughs, and then twists her mouth, have her cough, twist her mouth, and then blink. If she typically swings her right arm, have her swing her left.

6. *Generalization. In Class.* Make each teacher who works with the student aware of her fluency rule. They then can assist the student with monitoring her in-class compliance with this rule when she reads aloud, discusses, asks a question, or provides an answer. *At Home.* Have the student's parents hang a full-length mirror in her room. The mirror can be used for massed practice assignments and to monitor associated behaviors while reading aloud or talking on the telephone. *Community Experience.* Have the student go into a clothing store with a friend and request a particular brand of blue jeans in her size. Have her friend observe for any associated behaviors.

CHAPTER 10 /
OTHER DYSFLUENCIES

33. CLUTTERING

DETECTION Watch for students who display:

- Rapid rate of speech
- Absence of pauses so that words crowd each other
- Slurred articulation
- Ability to speak clearly when asked to do so
- Unawareness of having a speech problem

Description. *Cluttering* is a disorder of the timing in speech. It is a type of rapid, indistinct, and staccato utterance that can become unintelligible at times. The speaker delivers the words at a fast rate, called *tachylalia*, which increases as he speaks. The words rush out and fall upon each other without the temporal spacing that normally separates one from another. Phrasing is abnormal, with the speaker pausing in the middle of a sentence segment to catch a breath; sentence structure may be disorganized as well. The listener must work hard to follow the thought as the speaker continues at top speed, omitting sounds and syllables or telescoping words. Articulation and intelligibility suffer as speed increases. Some clutterers confuse the verbal barrage even more by interjecting extra syllables, such as "uh," "well," or "hmn," or by repeating an entire phrase. The repetition is very different from that of a stutterer; it is not an effort to get past a juncture of the sentence but more an attempt to fill every moment with sound. It appears to be a compulsive repetition that may occur in the middle of the sentence or at the end. For instance, the clutterer may say, "I'm going outside, going outside to play," or "I'm going outside to play, to play." There is no break in fluency, and the speaker seems to be unaware of the repetition.

Causation. Strangely, the clutterer usually can speak perfectly well for a brief time when asked to do so. Cluttering is referred to by some as a syndrome that includes disordered speech, since it has been observed that other motor patterns are also rapid and sometimes imprecisely performed. Walking and eating are often hurried, as are the language arts of writing and reading. It has been noted that many persons with cluttering speech have family members with similar rapid speech and/or motor patterns. Some cluttering is evidently relatively common in children, since so many are brought to the attention of speech pathologists with the comment that "they talk too fast and chop up their words." Cluttering appears to be independent of intellectual level, as it is present in some individuals throughout the range of mental abilities.

Implications. There is some indication that early cluttering of speech may lead to stuttering behavior later. Both cluttering and stuttering are sometimes observed in the same speaker, while other persons who clutter never show any symptoms of stuttering. The most noticeable difference between cluttering and stuttering is that the clutterer seems unaware that his speech is abnormal in any way. Although the clutterer is often asked to repeat, he does not become self-conscious nor does he appear to develop tension and fear of speaking. Treatment should include efforts to help the clutterer become more aware of his speech pattern, monitor his own speech, and assume more responsibility for successful communication with others.

CORRECTION Modify these strategies according to the student's learning style, needs, and age.

1. *Self-Appraisal.* Tape record the clutterer speaking spontaneously; play the tape back in private and ask the student for comments about rate and intelligibility. Tape record another speaker using normal speech rate. Guide the target student to compare the number of words per minute and then the number of repetitions. Discuss the differences in the recordings.
2. *Their Appraisal.* Tape record the clutterer reading aloud (begin after the first 100 words) for 3 minutes. Have the speaker submit the tape to 10 friendly listeners who will rate his speech on a 1–10 scale of intelligibility. This is an important step for the student to become aware of deviant speech. Determine the severity of the problem together.
3. *Slow Down.* Tape record the clutterer reading aloud after instructions to "slow down and speak very distinctly." (Begin taping when the student starts reading.) Compare 3 minutes of this tape with the previous tape.
4. *Ta Tum, Ta Tum.* Ask the clutterer to read (easy reading material) with an imposed rhythm of unaccented syllable, accented syllable, repeated throughout the selection. Demonstrate the technique and then read with the student initially.
5. *Hear the Beat.* Tape record a steady beat (a wooden handle on a book cover produces a nice sound) and play as background while the student reads for 3 minutes. This even measure provides a reminder to help prevent progressive acceleration.
6. *Verse to Better.* Choose several selections of poetry with strong iambic meter (unstressed/stressed) for the student to memorize for oral presentation at a normal speech rate. Help the student to develop appropriate expression and tempo.
7. *Show Down.* Devise a graphic system of recording performance over individual trials. As the student reads new material, record each time the listener cannot understand a word or notes the insertion of irrelevant sounds or words. Keep a chart to show the speaker how the cluttering delivery has changed over time.
8. *Once Is Enough.* Ask the student to speak spontaneously, choosing from suggested topics such as My Favorite TV Program, What I Do/Don't Like about School, or What I Did Last Weekend. Tape record the student talking for 3–4 minutes. Later play the tape while both you and the student listen and mark the number of times words or phrases are repeated.

34. SITUATIONAL DYSFLUENCY

DETECTION Watch for students who display:

- Variability over time in occurrence of dysfluencies
- Absence of struggle behavior before phonation
- Frustration rather than anxiety while speaking

Description. *Dysfluency* is a common speech behavior that becomes an abnormality only when it occurs with unusual frequency and is accompanied by certain other behaviors. All speakers produce dysfluent speech at some time without it becoming a disability. Any break in the normal flow of speech could be called a dysfluency (literally, "impaired flow"). A speaker may pause between words, insert vocal fillers ("uh," "mmn") or phrases ("you know," "and then"), or repeat whole words or phrases.

Causation. Most children exhibit normally dysfluent speech during their early lan- guage-learning years. This typically occurs near the third year in the average child because this is generally a time of exposure to many new experiences and rapid cognitive growth. Often the child appears to have formed concepts before learning the words to express them, or she may want to ask questions without knowing the appropriate labels for the objects or actions. Dysfluent speech results as the child searches her small vocabulary, trying first one word and then another in her attempt to communicate adequately. In an effort to hold a busy adult's attention, the child may interject extraneous syllables or repeat words while she searches for a more suitable one. This word search may peak again at about age 5–6 as the child enters a structured school situation and has many more experiences to relate to significant others at home. During times of excitement or emotional stress, speakers of any age may become temporarily dysfluent. When the human nervous system is attending to unusual stimuli and formulating mental, physical, and physiological responses, the speech/language function of the brain appears to become less efficient. Verbal output may be marked by frequent pauses, irrelevant interjections, word searching, repetition of phrases, or other dysfluencies. When an individual is ill or becoming so and general physical vitality is low, speech production again may become disordered and inefficient. Many older people complain that they cannot recall a specific verbal label easily and their speech may reveal long pauses, nonword space fillers, and circumlocutions as they attempt to complete an utterance without the specific desired word. Certain diseases or traumas can have an effect on speech, either through dysfunction of the normal coordination of the speech mechanism or by interference with reception, organization, or other language processes.

Implications. While dysfluency interferes with smooth speech production, the listener often unconsciously adjusts expectations to account for the age, situation, and condition of the speaker. Therefore, the speech may be viewed as somewhat different than that produced by most speakers but not abnormal. Situational dysfluency derives from an inadequate vocabulary or the emotional or physical condition of the speaker and will change as that condition changes. If the stress is temporary, speech production will usually return to its previous level of competence; if the speaker has suffered a permanent physical impairment, then speech production may continue to be dysfluent. Listeners should attempt to assure the speaker that her communicative efforts are valued for their content and that she has whatever time she needs to complete her statement.

CORRECTION Modify these strategies for the student's learning style, needs, and age.

1. *Reinforcement.* When a student exhibits dysfluent speech, give her your attention; if feasible, pause in your activity to demonstrate that you are ready to listen to her message.
2. *Subtle Intervention.* A student who sometimes talks in a halting or repetitious manner should be encouraged to speak more smoothly by indirect approaches. The speech should not be labeled stuttering, nor should the child become the center of anxious attention because of the broken flow of speech.
3. *Cool It.* A speaker who is temporarily dysfluent may improve when the listener exhibits a quiet, supportive manner. This listening attitude may provide a calming influence and reduce the speaker's anxiety, so that a smoother flow of speech is possible.
4. *Help Me.* Older persons or those who have sustained a brain injury of some type may experience less frustration if the listener assists their word searching pauses by suggesting words to them. Observation of the speaker's reaction to this should indicate how much help is welcome.
5. *Study-Up.* Some students appear to be dysfluent at school, although the behavior is not observed in other situations. It is possible that a lack of phonic skills and unfamiliarity with vocabulary may be the basic problem. The student, when reading aloud, may display frequent pauses, as well as repetitions of parts of or whole words. This speech pattern may become generalized to all academic recitations. Thorough teaching of vocabulary with frequent reviews before the student reads orally may produce a smoother production.
6. *Redirection.* Persons whose dysfluency is apparently connected to stress caused by conflict, anxiety, or fear centering on a specific situation may produce normally fluent speech when they turn their attention to other areas of their lives. They may be helped by a listener who will unobtrusively redirect the conversation to less stressful topics.
7. *Word Support.* It should be helpful to dysfluent speakers who have difficulty finding the appropriate words for their thoughts to have a time for review of the vocabulary most troublesome for them. Parents of young children can attempt to provide the youngsters with words to express their feelings, to describe novel experiences, and to name new objects with which they come in contact.

REFLECTIONS

1. Stuttering has been reported among various cultural groups down through recorded time. From your understanding of the disorder as discussed in Chapter 9, state whether you think it is caused by physiological or psychological factors. Be prepared to defend your opinion with examples, statistics, or other source materials.

2. Various aspects of stuttering are presented in Chapter 9; which of them (repetition, prolongation, hesitation, speech blocks, or associated symptoms do you consider most characteristic of stuttering as you understand it? Do you think this is the most distracting aspect?

3. A speech pathologist who wishes to help a person who stutters should first attempt to understand the speaker's feelings. It is frequently suggested that one should adopt the stuttering speech to use during a verbal exchange with a stranger in order to experience the reaction of listeners to stuttered speech. Do you think this is a good idea? What benefits could there be? Could there be negative effects? Explain your viewpoint.

4. Dysfluent speech can be very disconcerting to the speaker. Have you ever felt that your speech was abnormally dysfluent? What was the speaking situation and why do you think you were dysfluent at that time? How would you describe your feelings then?

5. To accommodate a severe stutterer in the regular classroom, a teacher must be aware of some basic principles. If one of the students in your fourth-grade class was a severe stutterer, how would you adjust your requirements for class participation or what other steps would you take to alleviate the student's embarrassment? List five specific actions you would take.

6. Occasionally, one hears of a person with normal speech who suddenly begins stuttering after an emotional shock or a student who begins stuttering in imitation of another person's speech. Do you feel that these stories are accurate? Be prepared to present arguments both in agreement with and in opposition to the stories.

7. Some persons with dysfluent speech exhibit a number of secondary behaviors. Review Skill 32 for a description of some distracting physical concomitants of the abnormal speech. Would you give attention first to the speech or to the accompanying physical activities? Defend your choice.

8. Some teachers recognize cluttering but do not understand it. As you talk with teachers, ask if they have had students who were difficult to understand because of a rapid speech rate. Do not use the word *clutter* but ask them to describe the student's speech pattern as fully as possible. Ask if the behaviors described in Skill 33 were noted in that student. Ask what efforts the teacher made to improve the student's speech.

9. Information in Chapter 9 describes repetitions, prolongations, hesitations, and speech blocks. Review these discussions and be prepared to demonstrate each of them for a peer. You will then be a listener while that person demonstrates the same stuttering speech patterns for you.

10. Some types of dysfluent speech are not considered to be true stuttering. Describe some of these. How do they differ from stuttering, and what therapeutic approach would you recommend for each?

11. Secondary behaviors accompanying stuttering may be related to several factors. Refer again to Skills 31 and 32; which of the secondary behaviors would you attribute to fear or anxiety affecting the speaker? Defend your choices.

12. There has been a great deal of research and many individuals have developed their own theories regarding the causes of dysfluent speech. As a result, treatment recommendations also vary widely. It should be of interest for the reader to compare and contrast the viewpoints expressed in these references with the information presented in Chapter 9.

Curlee, R. F., & Perkins, W. H. (1984). *Nature and treatment of stuttering: New directions.* San Diego, CA: College-Hill Press.

Fiedler, P. A., & Standop, R. (1983). *Stuttering: Integrating theory and practice.* Austin, TX: Pro-Ed.

Ingham, R. J. (1984). *Stuttering and behavior therapy: Current status and experimental foundations.* San Diego, CA: College-Hill Press.

Leith, W. R. (1984). *Handbook of stuttering therapy for the school clinician.* San Diego, CA: College-Hill Press.

McReynolds, L., & Spradlin, J. (1988). *Generalization strategies in the treatment of communication disorders.* St. Louis, MO: B. C. Decker.

Peins, M. (1984) *Contemporary approaches in stuttering therapy.* San Diego, CA: College-Hill Press.

Prins, D., & Ingham, R. J. (1983). *Treatment of stuttering in early childhood: Methods and issues.* San Diego, CA: College-Hill Press.

Shames, G. H., & Rubin, H. (1986). *Stuttering: Then and now.* Columbus, OH: Charles E. Merrill.

Starkweather, C. W. (1987). *Fluency and stuttering.* Englewood Cliffs, NJ: Prentice-Hall.

Wells, B. (1987). *Stuttering treatment: A comprehensive clinical guide.* Englewood Cliffs, NJ: Prentice-Hall.

Winitz, H. (Ed.) (1989). *Human communication and its disorders. 1989 annual review* (Vol. 3). Norwood, NJ: Ablex.

PART V

LANGUAGE

The ability to communicate must begin with learning the system that is accepted by other members of one's social group. In our society, spoken language is the basic means of communication and it is through hearing speech that one normally learns how to use speech to interact with others. Language is used to communicate ideas, to give information, and to satisfy curiosity through questioning. It is a social tool that becomes more effective as the individual learns to employ it more proficiently. Language has a vocabulary, or lexicon, that the group has agreed has more or less specific meaning. In addition, certain grammatical regularities should be observed. These regularities, or rules of grammar, are usually learned by induction. The young child, through trial and error as well as comparison with mature speech patterns, learns to apply the rules of a native language without having consciously thought about it. Unfortunately, some students do not easily acquire the same facility with language that their peers enjoy. Their problem is not the production of speech sounds but their ordered deployment into a stream of connected speech that accurately conveys ideas and information.

Chapters 11 through 13 examine the areas of verbal language governed by rules. These three divisions—semantics, morphology, and syntax—cannot really be separated since each one is a part of and is influenced by the others.

However, in order to highlight skills in each area, these aspects are treated separately in this book.

The topic of Chapter 11, "Semantics," concerns the meaning assigned to words, an area of confusion for some students. Meaning can vary according to the level of abstraction and the specificity of vocabulary. Multiple meanings and figurative language expressions vary with the cultural backgrounds and experiences of the speakers; expressions from the past may fade into disuse while fresh, colorful language springs from ethnic groups, technological changes, or new life-styles. The concepts of space, time, and cause/effect require rapid mental manipulation of ideas before the meaning becomes clear. Prepositions are small words that the language-impaired student may overlook or misinterpret, thereby altering the meaning of a verbal message.

"Morphology," Chapter 12, concerns the use of morphemes, the smallest unit of speech to carry meaning. Morphemes often occur at the ends of words, are unstressed, and therefore may be overlooked. Comparisons denote differences in amount of a specific quality and may or may not require an -er or -est ending. Other areas of uncertainty for some students are the use of singular and plural forms, correct case and gender, personal pronouns, verbs, and verb phrases.

The third major component of verbal language to be considered is syntax in Chapter 13. Syntax refers to the order in which words are arranged. This section is of special importance to those working with students who seem to lose their way in sentences that contain clauses, phrases, or anything but noun-verb-object sentence order. Comprehension and use of complex sentences as well as techniques of questioning are essential classroom skills in most every subject area. Perhaps the most important of all the syntax skills is that of sequencing. A deficiency is easily noticed, and the underlying disability causes difficulty at the semantic and morphological levels as well.

Chapter 14 addresses word-finding difficulties. These include the disruption of recall ability in such areas as associations and categorization. Circumlocutions, characteristic of most speakers upon occasion but problematic when they occur too often, are also discussed.

Chapter 15 describes two special language problems: echolalia and delayed language. Echolalia is an outward manifestation of failure to achieve inner organization. Delayed language is not a disorder but a problem of slow development with the likelihood of some limitation of linguistic achievement in adulthood. Students in both groups present unique problems and challenges as they try to communicate in a highly verbal world.

Chapter 16, the final chapter, reminds the reader of the nonverbal communication skills that enhance and enliven all interpersonal exchanges.

It is important to remember that a language-impaired student may not need to learn all the skills presented in this part. Teachers and speech pathologists must analyze each student's present level of competence, probable level of future achievement, and the need for certain skills and then prioritize the time allotted so that the most essential skills will be mastered.

35. MULTIPLE MEANINGS

DETECTION Watch for the student who:

- Produces a single interpretation of multiple-meaning words
- Has a sparse receptive and expressive vocabulary
- Misunderstands idioms and figurative language

Description. This task requires the student to be able to interpret dual meaning words in more than one way. Language-disordered children and youth may focus on a single meaning of a word that has multiple meanings. For example, if the student defines *glasses* only as "spectacles," then he may have a great deal of difficulty understanding why his mother asked him to "put the glasses in the dishwasher."

Causation. Single interpretation of multiple-meaning words may stem from difficulties understanding abstractions. Students may prefer word meanings that are more concrete, have a relatively high frequency of occurrence in the language, and with which they have had personal experiences.

Implications. Students who are unable to interpret dual-meaning words in more than one way will experience much difficulty in the academic arena and in interpersonal relationships. Difficulties are likely to arise in the following academic areas: reading, literature, composition, social studies, science, and foreign languages. Interpersonal relationships will likely suffer from impaired communication.

CORRECTION Modify these strategies for the student's learning style, needs, and age.

1. *Dictionary Match-Up.* Assemble pictures that represent multiple-meaning words. Print short dictionary definitions (from a dictionary used in the lower-elementary grades) on 3" x 5" cards. The student will match the dictionary definition to the pictorial representation. The difficulty level of this activity can be altered by varying the number of selections from which the student chooses the definition and the number of pictures to be defined.

Sample words:

state	plum	trim
diner	short	turn
fool	pink	coin
telephone	beat	suit
light	pose	bear
print	glasses	tax

2. *"I'll Have a Light."* Create a commercial like the Bud Light beer commercial which illustrates the dangers of nonspecific communication. In the commercial a customer in a bar orders a "light." Instantly a ring of fire with poodles jumping through the ring appears, or a Fourth of July fireworks display erupts, or a match is struck and a cannon is ignited. The customer realizes his error and then asks for the specific brand of light beer. The point of the commercial is that there are multiple meanings of the word *light*. Discuss why the commercial is effective and entertaining.

3. *Double Duty.* Present sentences that have multiple interpretations. The student will give at least 2 interpretations of each sentence.

Sample sentences:

He wiped the glasses.
The sailor kept the watch.
The woman did not press the suit.
Please describe the victim's state.
The minister married the young couple.
The teenager wore a loud shirt.
Pick your friends carefully.
Dad smoked the turkey for Thanksgiving dinner.
The pitcher burned the ball across the plate.
The teacher questioned the student pointedly.

4. *Riddlemania.* Find an old riddle book and present certain riddles to the students. Have the students explain the humor in each riddle.

Sample riddles:

- Q: Why did the little boy put his father in the refrigerator?
  A: He wanted cold pop.
- Q: Why did the little boy throw his clock out of the window?
  A: He wanted to see time fly.
- Q: When is a boy not a boy?
  A: When he turns into a store.
- Q: What is the best way to keep a skunk from smelling?
  A: Hold its nose.
- Q: Which will burn longer: the candles on the birthday cake of a boy or the candles on the birthday cake of a girl?
  A: No candles burn longer. They all burn shorter.

5. *Cloze Rebus.* Using the pictures in Activity 1, create a story (or use the one presented below) in which certain words have been omitted. Present the 2 pictures to cloze the sentence. The student will select the picture that gives the appropriate meaning.

Dinner for One

The old (fool) entered the (diner). He sat down and looked at the water (glasses). "These (glasses) are beautiful," he said. "Sure (beats) any I've got at home. They (suit) me just fine." He ate his meal and paid for it with a silver (coin).

36. FIGURATIVE LANGUAGE

DETECTION Watch for the student who:

- Displays poor comprehension in reading
- Fails to appreciate verbal humor
- Fails to understand multiple meanings
- Misses implied meanings

Description. This use of figures of speech requires the student to understand multiple meanings and to associate one event with another as a means of description. Figurative language requires flexibility in manipulating concepts and is based upon visual images. It is far more difficult to deduce the intended meaning when the words are not to be taken at face value. The reader or listener must become an active participant in the communication event. Many culturally different students are familiar with figurative language in their own culture but do not have the cognitive or experiential foundation to understand the figurative comparisons made in their reading books or in classroom discussions and examples.

Causation. Difficulties with this abstract use of language may arise from a limited vocabulary, in which case the student simply does not know the word or the specific intended meaning. Limited experience accounts for some failures to understand figures of speech. "Like a bull in a china shop" means little to a student who has seen neither a bull nor a china shop. In fact, to her, *bull* may be a slang expression and *china* a foreign country. A student who has not advanced beyond the concrete stage of conceptualization will not appreciate the subtleties of figurative language. "Give me your heart" or "He asked for her hand in marriage" could horrify that child. Phrases such as "An iron fist in a velvet glove" make little sense to some students without teacher explanation. A lack of imagination may interfere with the formation of mental pictures to illustrate the words. Imagination flourishes when cultivated but withers when discouraged. Some youngsters come to school without the advantage of early exposure to the fanciful characters and plots found in children's stories. While some children live in language-poor homes, where speech seldom goes beyond basic communication, other homes are rich in idioms and similes that are an integral part of everyday conversation. In both cases, however, the students may never have heard the figures of speech they encounter in the classroom.

Implications. Students who have difficulty in this area will have poor comprehension for poetry and for some stories. This may become apparent after the third grade, at which point reading material begins to contain more figurative language. The student may be able to read all the words but not be able to follow the thoughts because of a phrase or allusion that seems extraneous. "George, bulldog that he was, remained at the door" may translate to the student as "George's bulldog remained at the door" and create confusion in the storyline. Such a student will not easily handle references to those persons who "glide," "sail," or "slip" into a room or others who "storm," "thunder," and "explode." In social interaction, these individuals often miss the points of jokes and do not quite seem to understand the quick exchange of humorous remarks.

CORRECTION Modify these strategies according to the student's learning style, needs, and age.

1. *Preteach.* Before the student reads a selection, the teacher can extract the instances of figurative language and explain the usage of the words. It is better to prevent confusion than to try to dispel it.
2. *Word Search.* Cultivate abstract thinking in the student through lessons on choosing descriptive words. Begin with the concrete, and help the student to move on to more abstract conceptions. A hummingbird may be described as "green," "a blur of color," or "a tiny helicopter." Students might begin with descriptive words for animals or for verbs (running, eating, laughing). It might be helpful to enact the words and let the students develop the abstraction (lumbering, gobbling, roaring) or "like an elephant," "inhaling his food," and "choked with laughter."
3. *Sense-Able Lessons.* Use sensory experiences to stimulate a student's ability to use descriptive language. Bring objects for observing, tasting, feeling, hearing, and smelling, and then compile a list of the students' verbal reactions. A classroom Halloween party, with the subjects blindfolded as they touch peeled grapes; taste a "witch's brew"; hear moans, howls, and shrieks; accompanied by the smell of burning leaves will be fun for teacher and students. These vivid sensations will trigger descriptive abilities and help students to comprehend the mental imagery of others.
4. *Explain That.* Prepare a list of idioms in common usage and discuss them in class. Help the students to discover the connection between the given words and their actual meanings. These examples can start the list:
   - He had a green thumb. (Thumbs are used to press dirt around plant roots thereby helping the plant to grow well and stay green.)
   - She had two left feet. (Two left feet would cause one to be awkward.)
   - He was on pins and needles. (This would be an uncomfortable position which he would be eager to change.)
   - They were walking on eggs. (They were carefully trying to prevent a probable disagreeable situation.) Encourage the students to add other idioms to your list.
5. *As-a-Zoo.* Help students to recognize similes they use or have heard. Mention some common phrases and explain that they really are comparisons between 2 things:

As quiet as a mouse	As free as a bird
As slow as a turtle	As snug as a bug in a rug
As hungry as a horse	As sly as a fox
As slippery as a fish	As timid as a rabbit

37. SPACE AND TIME RELATIONSHIPS

DETECTION Watch for the student who:
- Cannot express future or past time adequately
- Cannot comprehend units of distance and measurement

Description. Some language-disabled students have difficulty discussing events that do not take place here and now. Their conception of the future and past is unclear as is their understanding of distance. Such a student speaks of anything past as "a long time ago," even if it was last week, but events that occurred several years ago may be differentiated as "a long, long time ago." One language-disabled student was heard to say that he was going to his grandmother's house to stay "one night, and another night, and another night." He did not know how to describe it as "a weekend." These students seem to live in an unstructured timeframe and have not assimilated the progressively larger units of time. They often have difficulty understanding how the time units of days, weeks, months, and years relate to one another. The notion of time being fluid (e.g., today becomes yesterday and the future dissolves into present and past) confuses them. Distance is equally abstract, so the terms used in measuring distance become confused with one another. As a further complication, relativity enters in, so that what is *near* in one context may be *far* in another (e.g., a student's home is near the school, yet it is too far from school to walk home in bad weather). The student must also attempt to make sense of variable terms such as *now, later, before, soon, to town, to the store, to work,* and *to the lake.*

Causation. A student who is a concrete thinker learns *up* as it applies to his movement in space and later *down.* When he encounters these words in relation to other objects and events, he may become confused. A deficit in the central nervous system sometimes causes a student to be unsure of his own location in space in relation to chairs, tables, and doors. Presumably, this confusion extends to everything in the visual field and is multiplied when the student is asked to order space that cannot be seen. The language-disabled student finds it difficult to understand and use terms that shift in meaning.

Implications. This student is apt to have difficulty organizing events in space and time, which will cause problems in all academic areas. Conventional usage of prepositions may develop slowly and may need to be overlearned before becoming automatic. Abstract terms of time or spatial relationships should be illustrated with several examples. Pictures, maps, graphs, and timelines are helpful in relating events and places.

CORRECTION Modify these strategies for the student's learning style, needs, and age.

1. *Turn About.* Help young children learn ordinal numbers by finding their place in line when they are assigned, first, second, third, and so on positions. Ask who is last in line; have the students turn around and then ask who is last. Identify the new first, second, third, and other ordinal positions.

2. *Measure.* Measure objects in the classroom and make a bulletin board that tells that the door, for example, is 5-1/2 feet high, the desk is 3 feet wide, the dictionary is 8 inches by 10 inches, and the room is 8 yards long. State the equivalents in feet and inches when applicable. Discuss how many miles it is from school to familiar places, such as a church, the post office, a shopping area, or a movie theater. The purpose of this exercise is to help students understand relative sizes and distances. It is suggested that instruction include the metric system only in areas where that system is widely used.

3. *Timeline.* Construct a timeline on the chalkboard with "Now" as the center point. Label the line to the right "Future" and the section to the left "Past." On the line, place "Tomorrow, Next Day" to the immediate right of the center, and "Yesterday, Last Night" to the left. Next, add "Next Week" and "Next Month," as well as "Last Week" and "Last Month." Write the names of the months in the appropriate places; ask students to tell where holidays and their birthdays should go. Discuss "a week ago, a month ago, long ago, ago," and where to place "after a while," later," "by and by," and other such phrases.

4. *What Time?* Teach words that indicate time by presenting them as new reading vocabulary. Write the words on the chalkboard with brief definitions; prepare pictures to illustrate each and ask the students to match the definitions to the given words. These examples may help you:

dawn	noon	twilight	afternoon
sunset	midnight	dusk	evening

5. *Calendar.* Provide sheets of paper marked in blocks for a calendar. Demonstrate for students how to label the month name, the days of the week, and the individual dates for that month. Then direct each student to choose events that will be important for him that month and write them on the spaces for the appropriate days. Events might include church, visit to friends, birthday party, spelling test, shopping, movie, piano lesson, scout meeting, or other activities. This should help students to learn to anticipate and prepare adequately for coming events.

6. *Follow My Map.* Provide students with sheets of graph paper marked with the largest squares available. Demonstrate how they can make a map to show the route from the classroom to the school office. Provide each student with gummed paper strips in 1-inch and longer lengths to use in marking the route. Approximate distances and emphasize the turns and the relative distances. Have students follow their own maps when they finish and then exchange maps with peers to confirm accuracy. Older students can then complete maps on the graph paper showing their route from home to school.

7. *Wake-Up.* Help younger children to begin to understand the concept of future time by teaching them to count the "wake-ups" until an event that is due to occur within 4–5 days. The event could be Friday, the school fair, library day, or any specific approaching activity.

8. *A-Mazing.* Create a simple maze in the classroom by arranging the desks in a new pattern for the students to walk through. After introductory trials, have them try it blindfolded. See how many students can draw a simple map of the maze pattern when it is not visible to them.

38. CAUSE/EFFECT RELATIONSHIPS

DETECTION Watch for the student who:
- Has difficulty answering "why" questions
- Sees causes and effects as separate events without connection
- Exhibits below-average ability to generalize

Description. Some students with language-learning problems may function adequately when receiving or using simple sentences but appear to have unusual difficulty with certain sentence constructions that require the mental manipulation of ideas. These students may comprehend cause and effect relationships when they are explicitly stated by another person but may be unable to formulate an original sentence stating an observed cause and effect. There may be difficulty both in recognizing the relationship and in stating it correctly.

Causation. This problem may have its roots in the failure to connect two events appropriately, such as "It was raining" and "I took my umbrella." The student might reason that the speaker took the umbrella first and fail to consider (or understand) the time constraint of the verb form in the first sentence. The student also might be confused by the vocabulary required; "I took my umbrella because it was raining" puts the effect before the cause, while "I took my umbrella since it was raining" is no better. Stating the cause before the effect produces "It was raining so I took my umbrella" and may be easier for the student to construct. Rigidity in thinking and a limited vocabulary may make this a more difficult concept to express than to understand.

Implications. The student who has difficulty comprehending and/or expressing cause and effect relationships is likely to experience problems in many academic areas. The analysis of reading selections requires the ability to recognize causes and effects in the storylines. Science certainly emphasizes the value of knowing "what causes this effect?" Social studies views human behavior as principally causes and effects and important predictions are based on recognizing the relationships.

CORRECTION Modify these strategies for the student's learning style, needs, and age.

1. *Get It Together.* Prepare slips of paper with either a cause or an effect written on them. Put 3–4 matched pairs of slips in an envelope and distribute to each member of a group. Ask students to make a sentence of the cause and effect and state it orally. The causes and effects could be similar to these:

Cause	Effect
I studied hard.	I made an A on the test.
He ate too much.	His stomach hurts.
Her hair was too long.	She cut her hair.
It rained all week.	The river flooded.

2. *Because.* Suggest causes to the students and ask them to imagine possible effects. You might want to begin with such causes as these:

The wind blew hard.	The shoes were too small.
He drove fast.	The wood got wet.
She took him a cake.	The price of oil went up.

3. *First Then.* Ask the students to produce original cause/effect sentences and use each of these words in the written statements: *because, therefore, so, as, since,* and the construction, "first _____, then _____."

4. *Walk About.* Take a walk around the schoolyard and ask the students to list as many effects and causes as they can. Notice such things as leaves on the ground, mudholes, trash, street conditions, sounds, weather conditions, and the like. After returning to the classroom, ask each student in turn to orally state an observed cause and effect.

5. *Why Ball.* Prepare a list of questions to ask students in the group. Ask the question, follow with a student's name, and toss a small ball to the student. The student must use *because* in a complete sentence in response and toss the ball back to the teacher. Accept any reasonable answer from the student. After a few practice rounds, wherein you model the procedures, try questions such as these:

Why do fish swim? Fish swim because they want to go someplace.

Why do dogs growl? Dogs growl because they are angry.

Why do boys get dirty? Boys get dirty because they play on the ground.

6. *If/Then.* Use the if/then construction to help students connect cause and effect. Begin with very easy and obvious examples and help students verbalize the relationships. Then present these partial statements and direct students to respond in complete oral statements:

If there were no clocks, then . . .

If he did not feed his parakeet, then . . .

If it rains tomorrow, then . . .

If my tooth hurts, then . . .

If I had ten dollars, then . . .

If there were no roads, then . . .

7. *Fables.* Read fables or stories with strong morals to the group; then discuss the outcome of each. Help students to remember the events that caused the story ending. Adjust the vocabulary and complexity of the stories to the ability levels of your students. Refer to Aesop's fables and folktales for ideas. Show filmstrips that teach lessons" and let students formulate statements concerning the observed causes and effects. These stories may be available in both book and filmstrip form:

"The Rabbit and the Turtle"

(The turtle kept walking, so it won the race.)

"The Fox and the Grapes"

(The fox could not get the grapes, so he said they were sour.)

"The Greedy Dog"

(The dog lost the meat because he tried to grab it from the reflection in the water.)

"The Boy Who Cried Wolf"

(He did not get help when he needed it because he had called for help as a joke too often.)

"The Grasshopper and the Ant"

(The grasshopper got hungry because he had not worked to store food for winter.)

39. PREPOSITIONAL PHRASES

DETECTION Watch for the student who:
- Confuses common prepositions
- Misunderstands directions containing prepositions

Description. The language-impaired student has more than usual difficulty learning to comprehend and use the simplest prepositions of location (e.g., *in, on, under*). It is even harder for that student to learn the prepositions with uncertain location, such as *over, by, above, in front of,* and *next to* (which at some point becomes *away from*). That student never is sure whether the boat is *in* the water or *on* the water and whether the car is *in* or *on* the street. The language-disabled student may have extreme difficulty understanding that the same nut can be *beneath* the tree *on* the hill *under* a leaf *on* the ground *by* a hole. Confusion concerning location, direction, or time, as stated by prepositional phrases, may cause the student to ignore the phrases used by others and to rely on indefinite descriptors (e.g., *over there, that one, there, sometime*) in his own speech.

Causation. This is one aspect of a general disability for comprehending verbal communication. It may relate to the student's lack of attention to the unstressed words of sentences. It seems that language-impaired students may continue to depend on the subject, verb, and object or adverb to carry the meaning of the sentence, as they did when they were younger. The problems result from a failure to adjust their decoding approach to increased linguistic demands. These students appear to have fewer strategies for organizing information, so confusion mounts when sentences become longer.

Implications. Students who do not attend to or understand prepositional phrases will be at a disadvantage in following and giving explicit directions. To facilitate the student's growth in comprehension and his use of prepositional phrases, unfamiliar prepositions should be introduced and specifically taught in advance of their inclusion in classroom lessons. It is important for students to learn to decode all the words in sentences, particularly if they are to succeed at academic subjects at advanced levels. Comprehension must precede the ability to use prepositional phrases with sufficient precision to meet the communicative requirements of classroom tasks and many vocations as well.

CORRECTION Modify these strategies for the student's learning style, needs, and age.

1. *Ball Game.* Teach young children simple prepositions of location by changing the position of a small ball in relation to an open box. Have the child place the ball in, on, under, by, over, in front of, in back of, away from, and against the box. For each position, state, "The ball is ____ the box," and ask the child to repeat the statement. Then teacher or child can ask, "Where is the ball?" for the other to reply.

2. *Draw-a-Picture.* Give students drawing paper and pencils and instruct them to draw a picture as you describe it. Instructions might include:

> Draw a house; put a tree beside the house. Put a ladder against the tree. Put a squirrel on the house. Put a bird over the tree. Put 2

apples on the tree and 1 apple under the tree. Draw a lake behind the house. Put a boat on the lake. Put 2 men in the boat. Draw a cat between the house and the tree. Make flowers in front of the house. Make a fence go around the flowers.

When the pictures are finished, have the students take turns describing them while you check to see if everyone understood all the prepositions. Then have students sign their pictures in the corner and display them on the classroom wall.

3. *Exercise.* Play an exercise game by asking students to stand and follow your rhyming directions:

Put your hands on your head,
Put your thumbs on your toes,
Stick your fingers in your ears,
Put your left wrist on your nose.
Hold your hands behind your back,
Drop your chin down to your chest,
Stick your tongue way out in front,
Come on, now, do your best!
Put your hands on your shoulders,
Touch your elbow to the floor,
Put one foot behind the other,
Don't give up, we'll do some more.
Put your hands between your knees,
Make your eyes go up and down,
Put your thumbs beneath your chin,
While you turn right and right around!

4. *Is It One?* Explain to the students that some words function as more than 1 part of speech, according to how they are used. Warn them that what looks or sounds like a preposition may not always be a preposition. Use the words in sentences in which they will sometimes be used as prepositions and sometimes not. Write them on separate slips of paper for each student to sort into "Preposition" and "Not a Preposition" stacks.

Words: like, out, down, off, through, up
I like to read. I read books like that.
He went out the door. The boy struck out.
Put the pencil down. She lives down the street.
It fell off the roof. Please turn the water off.
Are we through for today? Did it go through the pipe?
The airplane went up. The teacher ran up the steps.

5. *Finish It.* Tell the students that you will start an oral sentence that they are to finish with a prepositional phrase. Demonstrate by allowing volunteers to finish a few sentences; then ask each student in turn to finish a sentence such as:

He fell _____.   They went _____.
She ate lunch _____.   The lady put the books _____.
Angel gave it _____.   Alison called him _____.
The ball rolled _____.   The teacher talked _____.

CHAPTER 12

MORPHOLOGY

40. COMPARATIVES

DETECTION Watch for the student who:

- Uses comparatives and superlatives inconsistently or incorrectly
- Does not understand the rule of two or more
- Uses -er and -est endings on irregular forms

Description. Students who are language disabled commonly have deficiencies in understanding and using the adjectives or adverbs which denote comparison between two objects (comparative form) and comparison among more than two objects (superlative form). They also sometimes have difficulty understanding which adjectives and adverbs do not require the -er and -est endings. Such students frequently restrict the use of those descriptive adjectives and adverbs of which they are uncertain and overuse a few basic words that they have mastered.

Causation. Most linguistically handicapped students have a history of difficulties with language that usually began before they spoke their first words. They have struggled to communicate, they have attempted to remember vocabulary, they have finally achieved some success with syntactical constructions—and then morphological endings are brought to their attention. It appears that, after having surmounted major difficulties, the student is not concerned about precise endings on certain words. If the meaning is communicated to the listener, the language-impaired student may not be highly motivated to improve.

Implications. An uncertainty concerning the choice of comparative or superlative endings for adjectives and/or adverbs may not be of major importance to the language impaired speaker. However, the use of incorrect forms, such as *mostest, bestest,* or *beautifulest,* mark the speaker as immature or uneducated. Such usage can create not only academic but also social problems and would certainly interfere with success in most adult situations.

CORRECTION Modify these strategies for the student's learning style, needs, and age.

1. *Speak Quickest.* Display several objects to the class and point out their relative roundness, hardness, smallness, or other attributes. Guide students to compare the objects and verbalize their comparisons. Try naming other items in groups of 3 and let the students respond. Then tell the group that they are to listen closely and call out the answer as soon as they can but they can answer only once. The student who responds correctly first gets candy or other reward placed on a tissue on her desk. Name 3 objects, then ask the question.

Rock, pillow, apple: Which is the softest?
Garbage, chair, lemon: Which is the smelliest?
Sidewalk, grass, ice: Which is the slickest?
Dollar, quarter, plate: Which is the flattest?
Straw, cocoa, wood: Which is the brownest?
Water, honey, oil: Which is the thickest?

As a variation of the activity, these groups of 3 objects can also be arranged from least to most, as in, "Arrange these items from least soft, to softer, to softest: rock, pillow, lemon."

2. *In Order.* Instruct the students in the use of the *-est* ending when comparing 3 or more items; then reinforce with this game. Prepare small rectangles from file folders by writing a series of words related by some characteristic. Place them in envelopes and pass an envelope to each student. At the signal to begin, the student will take out the rectangles and arrange them in order according to the instruction on the front of the envelope. These are examples:

smallest to largest (bug, bird, dog, horse)
largest to smallest (elephant, cow, pig, mouse)
loudest to quietest (fire alarm, yell, doorbell, whisper)
shortest to tallest (match, straw, broom, fence, telephone pole)
hottest to coldest (sun, boiling water, apple, ice cream)
smoothest to roughest (silk, wool, corduroy, snakeskin)
oldest to youngest (grandmother, mother, teenager, baby)

For younger or less able students, use pictures and give the directions orally.

3. *Going Shopping.* Divide your group into 2 teams of shoppers. Provide a copy of a comprehensive catalog to each team for reference as needed. Tell Team 1 they are to buy the cheapest of 3 items named and Team 2 is to buy the costliest item. Individual players, 1 from each team, are to respond orally as soon as they can. The player to answer correctly first by saying "The _____ costs least" or "The _____ costs most" wins a point. The team with the most points wins. Conceal the words while you are writing them on a transparency and display them all at the same time. These examples should get you started:

house, horse, hamburger
pen, purse, panda
book, bandage, bed
curtain, candy bar, carpet
knife, nut, nail polish
jacket, jelly, Jaguar

4. *Class Act.* Relate a simple story that tells of 3 boys (tall, taller, tallest) who went fishing and got (wet, wetter, wettest) while catching fish (big, bigger, biggest); their mother put on an apron and fixed soup and salad for them. As you tell the story, give the first adjective or adverb, and then point to the group to supply the comparative and superlative forms. Incorporate into the story additional comparatives, such as *fast, tiny, red, round, sour, sweet, hot, juicy, pretty, good,* and *sleepy.*

41. NUMBER

DETECTION Watch for students who:

- Omit final "s" on plural nouns when needed
- Add final "s" on nouns when not needed
- Omit final "s" on active verbs
- Have difficulty with subject-verb number agreement

Description. Some students appear to be confused as to the proper usage of final "s." They may say, "Two bird fly away" and later, "I saw some mens in the yard." Nouns that end in "s" may acquire another "es," as in *pantses* while the irregular plural form *feet* may be ignored in favor of *foots.* The active-tense verb in the third-person singular often is used without the final "s," as in "He run," "She say OK," or "The cat sit by the fire."

Causation. Some immature students habitually drop the final "s," as do some mentally handicapped students. It seems that their language development is still at the stage of concentrating on the content of the word without noticing the variation in the ending. This is similar to the language production of many normal children of 3 or 4 years of age. Older students who do not use final "s" may come from a culture in which this is standard usage and they have learned what they have heard. In other cases, the speech models may have been indistinct so that the child learning early language simply did not hear the final "s." Later, when attempting to remediate his usage, he overgeneralizes and adds an "s" inappropriately in some instances. Still other students appear to be lazy speakers and do not regard the addition of "s" to be of enough importance to make the extra articulatory effort.

Implications. The student who does not master the correct usage of final "s" will be regarded as speaking substandard English in most situations. This may interfere with his reading comprehension and written expression skills in school, and will be a definite detriment when he enters the job market and interviews for employment.

CORRECTION Modify these strategies for the student's learning style, needs, and age.

1. *Sammy Snake.* Demonstrate the production of "s" and emphasize the sound. Ask the student to produce a strong "s" as though "you are Sammy Snake." Count objects in pictured groups, such as 2 hats, exaggerating the final "s," and continue with 3 cups and the like. Use no pictures with irregular plurals, such as *men* or *deer.*

2. *Hiss or Buzz.* Explain that some plural words ending in "s" have a buzzing sound ("zz-z") instead of a hissing sound. Ask the students to imitate your exaggerated production of *peas, apples, roses, beans,* and others. Display pictures of groups of objects; ask the students in turn to place the pictures under the chalkboard heading of "Hissing" or "Buzzing" according to the final sound. Do not say the words for the students.

3. *Irregulars.* Teach the irregular plural nouns specifically by preparing an instructional bulletin board display that includes pictures of the following objects with the words written beneath the pictures:

feet	deer
men	sheep
women	pants
geese	fish
children	mice

    Leave the display on the bulletin board for at least 2 weeks and refer to it each day in a 5-minute minilesson.

4. *Clap for "S."* Teach the students to listen for the plural "s" by playing an audiotape previously prepared. Direct the students to clap for each sentence that contains a plural noun ending in "s." Mix sentences that do and do not contain plural nouns:

    The cats drank milk.
    The horse ran away.
    The shoes are dirty.
    She saw the stars.
    I dropped the glass.
    Put the cards away.
    He made a mess.
    The books are there.
    I want some juice.

5. *I Have Two.* Divide the group into 2 teams. The first member of Team 1 should say an original sentence beginning with "I saw a ____" and ending with a noun. The first member of Team 2 should say, "(First student's name) saw a ____, but I saw 2 ____s." If the plural form is correct, that team gets a point, and the player makes a new sentence for the next player on Team 1 to supply the plural. If the plural is not correct, the next player on Team 1 has the opportunity to supply the correct plural, win a point for the team, and provide the next sentence. Encourage the students to use difficult words in an effort to stump the opposing team and win points for their own team.

6. *Two B or Not Two B.* Young children can learn to listen for final "s" to denote more than 1 by playing this game. In a shallow box lid, display 2 of each of the following items:

block	basket (tiny)
bead	bear (tiny)
button	brush (small)
bow	butterfly (plastic)
bracelet	bubble gum
bean	ball (small)
bell	bone (toy)
balloon	box (tiny)

    Tell each student in turn to give you *block* or *blocks* or any of the items in the box. Direct the student to use both hands if he is getting more than 1 (to discourage his seeking visual cues after 1).

42. CASE AND GENDER

DETECTION Watch for the student who:
- Continues use of me as a subject pronoun after age 4
- Incorrectly uses pronouns when two are combined by *and*
- Uses pronouns inconsistently in other constructions

Description. When small children begin to talk, they often speak of themselves in the first person, using *me* as in, "Me want to go." The child who continues to use this incorrect form after the age of 4 gives warning that the correct use of pronouns is not going to be learned easily. The child appears to prefer to use the objective case of all pronouns and uses them in all positions. Admittedly, it is a difficult linguistic feat to be able to make an instantaneous choice in the middle of a statement between two pronouns that apply to the same person. When the child is first formulating sentences, the attention is on the message, not the form; but with increasing experience, the correct grammatical forms should appear.

Causation. Students with delayed language of whatever cause take longer to learn the proper use of pronouns, much as they are slower to learn all aspects of oral language. Their social environment may not model correct usage except for *I, she,* and *he* as subjects. Informal oral conversation often contains pronoun usage that is incorrect but socially accepted in many groups. Unfortunately, TV advertising and popular songs frequently use a nominative pronoun in place of an objective, as in, "Nothing can go wrong with my man and I" or "She saw John and I." Incorrect use of *who* for *whom* is common and few youngsters feel confident that they have chosen the correct pronoun even after consideration. Students must assimilate and coordinate conflicting information issued from home environments and from school instruction; this is especially difficult for the linguistically handicapped.

Implications. Correct pronoun usage should be taught gradually, beginning with *I, he, she,* and *we* as the subjects of sentences. Direct and repeated presentation of other pronouns is often necessary to help language-disabled students learn the usage with a minimum of confusion. Expecting these students to memorize the rules of grammar and apply them is usually a vain hope. They seldom have difficulty with comprehension of pronouns, but may use them with limited success themselves.

CORRECTION Modify these strategies for the student's learning style, needs, and age.

1. *Cover It Up.* Write sentences on the chalkboard with a name and a blank in either the nominative or objective case. Give the student a piece of poster board with which to cover the name; then direct her to read the sentence orally and fill in the correct pronoun. Give the student 1 of these choices: I/me; he/him; she/her; they/them; or we/us. Using the sample sentence "Jane and _____ went to the store," illustrate how each nominative pronoun will fit, changing the order of *Jane* and pronoun for *he, she, they,* and *we.* Using the sample

sentence "The girl gave the tickets to John and ____," show students the correct use of *me, him, her, them,* and *us.* Then ask students to volunteer to complete the sentences on the chalkboard.

2. *Red or Green?* Make poster board signs with the pronouns, *I, he, she,* and *we* lettered in red on one side, and the pronouns *me, him, her, us,* and *them* lettered in green on the reverse side. Place them in file folders so the lettering cannot be seen. Divide the group into 2 teams: first, one team acts out a given sentence and then members of the opposing team draw folders. If one of the pronouns can replace a noun in the sentence, that team member stands in front of the person portraying a noun or holds the object-noun with the sign displaying the correct pronoun. Each team gets a point for every pronoun correctly used and loses 2 points for each incorrectly used. These sentences fit the game:

> His mother gives the book to Steven. (she, it, him)
> Melissa (the speaker) stood in line by Don and Ron. (I, it them)
> Robert threw the ball to Anna. (he, it, her)
> The girls handed their pencils to Jason (the speaker). (they, them, me)
> Karen (the speaker) and Jennifer pointed to the chair where Jim sat.
>   (I, it, he)

Help the students act out 2–3 sample sentences before beginning to keep score. This exercise allows for mild physical activity and is entertaining as well.

3. *Folder Fun.* Prepare cards for each student by writing several sentences on paper and then mounting them in file folders. Each sentence should contain underlined nouns that can be replaced by pronouns. Write the appropriate pronoun for each blank on a rectangle cut from old file folders. Place the pronoun rectangles in a box for each student in turn to draw. The pronoun is to be placed on a noun in any sentence on the card or if it cannot be used correctly returned to the box. The student who replaces all the underlined nouns first wins the game. Demonstrate with an extra card how the game is to be played and then monitor students as they play, providing direct instruction as needed. These sentences are examples:

> Betty threw the ball to John. (she, it, him)
> Susan and I went home with Alison. (we, her)
> Kevin and Brandon ate the cake. (they, it)
> The man fed the dogs. (he, them)
> Mother gave the money to Rebecca and me. (she, it, us)

4. *Who or Whom?* On slips of paper, write sentences containing names of persons or words indicating persons as subjects or objects of the verb or of prepositions. Let each student draw a slip, read the sentence orally, and then turn the sentence into a question using either *who* or *whom* for the underlined noun. Help students understand the task by using sample sentences such as these and following with the question:

> Janice went to town. (Who went to town?)
> They gave the package to the boy. (They gave the package to whom?)
> She shared her lunch with Pat. (She shared her lunch with whom?)

43. TENSE, ASPECT, AND MOOD

DETECTION Watch for the student who displays:

- Uncertainty as to precise meaning of verb phrases
- Overuse of present active or present progressive tense
- Confusion about the stated time of action

Description. Many language-impaired students exhibit great confusion with the comprehension of verb tense (past, present, future), aspect (completed, habitual, repetitive), and mood (indicative, imperative, subjunctive). They do not appear to differentiate the future and the nonfuture in verb phrases such as "He will have been fishing" or "She could have been fishing." In order to participate in running conversation, they must abandon the effort to analyze each word in the verb phrase and thereby arrive at the specific meaning. Most listeners attain a certain level of automatic comprehension of phrases in their native language, but some language-impaired listeners seem unable to achieve this. They must unravel verb phrases word by word each time they are heard or simply take the meaning of the basic verb and hope for later clarification of the message.

Causation. Many linguistically handicapped students reveal deficient sequencing skills in a number of different areas. The comprehension or use of a verb phrase denoting future or past completed action requires a level of competence in word sequencing that the student may not have achieved. In addition, a clear understanding of relative time is necessary, but time and space relationships are another source of confusion for many language-impaired students. The tendency for these students to scan (auditorily or visually) a sentence to derive the general meaning may cause them to disregard the auxilliary words and absorb only the concept of the action. Although the students can demonstrate that they have received the total auditory or visual message at some level, they appear to attend only to those aspects that carry the greatest meaning for them. The difficulty they experience with sequencing skills, understanding time and space, and attention to detail all appear to be ramifications of the underlying problem, which is assumed to be the result of some irregularity of neural functioning.

Implications. The inability to comprehend and use tense markers correctly limits the efficiency of communication with others. Continued effort should be made to help students gain more familiarity with verb phrases. Repeated experience with the forms may lead to more facility and accuracy in their use, both receptively and expressively.

CORRECTION Modify these strategies for the student's learning style, needs, and age.

1. *Progressing.* Prepare small rectangles cut from file folders by writing a present progressive verb on each. Have students choose a rectangle in turn and use the verb in the sentence "Today the students are _____(talking)." Follow with the past tense by using the sentence "Yesterday the students _____

(talked)" and then the future with "Tomorrow the students will _____ (talk)."
Use both regular and irregular verbs:

saying	crying	walking
skipping	typing	doing
touching	humming	sitting
fighting	sleeping	running
eating	climbing	drinking
singing	writing	laughing
riding	flying	seeing
throwing	bringing	falling

2. *Irregulars.* After presentation of irregular verbs whose past tense and past participle change spelling, introduce and demonstrate this activity. Prepare a file folder by cutting a 1" x 3-1/2" window with a razor edge on one side of the folder, placing the window 1" down from the top of the folder and centered on that side. Tape the sides together and insert a sheet of paper with sentences spaced to be seen individually in the window as the sheet is moved up in the folder by an attached tab. The sentences will use a verb in other than present active tense. The student is to write the number of the sentence on another sheet of paper, along with the basic verb form for the verb in that sentence. Here are some sample sentences:

Guy ran down the hill.
Julie drank some water.
They flew in the airplane.
Angel sat on the floor.
The sun had shone all day.
Paco had drawn a horse.
The paper had been slid under the door.
All the flowers will have grown in my yard.
Tai had been bitten by a snake.
Nobody had read the book.

3. *Tense Out.* Explain the 3 principal parts of verbs, present tense, past tense, and past participle, and write several on the chalkboard to demonstrate the forms. Have students add to the examples. Direct the first student in the group to state a verb in present tense, as in "I am." The second student should follow with the past tense, "I was," and the third student is to give the past participle, "I have been." The next student will then state the first-person, present tense of any new verb, and the game will proceed as before. The teacher/therapist must listen carefully to identify errors as soon as they occur. A student who gives an incorrect verb form drops out of the game; the student who outlasts the others is the winner.

4. *Display.* On 3" x 5" index cards write in large letters, 1 word to a card, the present tense, past tense, and past participle of a number of verbs. Give each student the cards for 5–6 verbs, which have been shuffled into random order. Demonstrate with another set of verb cards how they are to be arranged, each verb with its forms in horizontal order on the desk or table. Give a signal for all students to begin at the same time; notice who finishes first. Check for correct arrangement before declaring that student the winner.

CHAPTER 13 /
SYNTAX

44. SENTENCE TRANSFORMATION

DETECTION Watch for the student who:

- Does not understand reversal of actor-object in passive sentences
- Does not use order in sentence to determine direct-indirect object
- Does not understand relationship of clauses to noun-verb

Description. Language-disabled students may have significant problems in learning to decode some syntactic constructions and even more problems if they attempt to use them. Their language usage is not disordered but they continue to exhibit delays in comprehending the rules of their native language. They appear to rely on the use of familiar structures and fail to gain competence with more varied syntax. These students follow the pattern of normal language development but appear to make little progress with the comprehension and use of more difficult sentence structures. They seem comfortable with the subject-verb-object word order while sentence transformations may baffle them. A passive-voice sentence, such as "The man was seen by the lady," may be scanned as "Man seen lady" and that message retained. Sentences with relative clauses, such as "The man who spoke to the class yesterday will be here tomorrow," may confuse instead of inform the student. The use of indirect objects in sentences, such as "Throw the boy outside a ball," adds more confusion while other constructions, such as noun complements, adverb clauses, and inverted sentence order, sometimes are incomprehensible.

Causation. Linguistically impaired students appear to have various areas of specific language disability that are apparent in the context of oral speech. It is not possible to determine exactly how their neurological systems function; but it does become apparent as their communication skills falter that disturbances are interfering with normal development. According to some sources, a sizable group of youngsters have an atypical neural organization, often genetically influenced, which results in language-learning deficiencies. They may have average potential for learning, but their mode of learning is different and less efficient.

Implications. As students progress in school, they may learn the content but become entangled in the language of discussion, oral and/or written. Often they participate in an interesting lesson in class and gain confidence as they follow the demonstration, the pictures, and other illustrations, only to fail miserably when asked to tell or write about the experience later. Perhaps the best way to help students understand the underlying meaning of a sentence is to practice changing it from one type of structure to others: from complex sentence to simple sentences or to questions.

CORRECTION Modify these strategies for the student's learning style, needs, and age.

1. *Transform.* Explain to the students that they do transform sentences in their day-to-day conversations without realizing what they are doing. Illustrate several transformations using this sentence:

    Kenny drove the car.
    Did Kenny drive the car?
    Kenny did not drive the car.
    The car was driven by Kenny.

    Give simple declarative sentences for the students to transform in turn: first, question form; second, negative statement; and third, passive form.

2. *Mix-Up.* Write a complex sentence on the chalkboard with the words in scrambled order; have the students work out the correct order as a group project. Repeat with several sentences until the students have developed some facility. Later, as a follow-up activity, have students compete to reconstruct sentences. Write the words to sentences on rectangles cut from old file folders. Put all the words for one sentence in an envelope. Distribute an envelop to each student and give a signal for all to begin putting the words in grammatical order. Watch to see who finishes first, but check to see if the sentence is correct before declaring the winner. Demonstrate the reconstruction of several sentences before starting contest. Try these sentences:

    The teacher hurried because he was late.
    Paul, the captain of the team, was the tallest player.
    Carolyn, who was studying, did not see her.
    The ball rolled out the door and down the hall.
    Mother gave Jorenda all the cookies.

3. *Paraphrase.* Introduce the class to some poetic sentences in which the word order varies from common usage. Help them to locate the subject, verb, and other sentence components. After practicing together on several sentences, begin an individual exercise. Ask students to rewrite sentences in their own words and signal as soon as they finish. Record the time each student required as you collect that paper. A goal should be to decrease the amount of time necessary to paraphrase the sentence. The student with the shortest time wins. Write sentences such as these on the chalkboard, on a transparency, or on sheets for each student:

    What a good boy am I!
    Into the pool of the hotel quickly went the diver.
    Behind the door crouched the cat quietly waiting for the rat.
    As he waved, the baby the girl saw dropped his spoon.
    After setting there all day, the package was delivered to the boy.
    This red rose to the beauty queen I'll take.

4. *Combine.* Demonstrate combining several short sentences into one longer sentence containing all the same information, such as in these examples:

    Janice went to the store. Janice was hungry. It was raining.
    Jason was tall. He went to school. He hit his head on the door.
    Joe is a football player. He plays the piano. He is big.
    The book was John's. The book fell in the mud. John was angry.

45. COMPLEX SENTENCES

DETECTION Watch for the student who:
- Uses run-on sentences and incomplete sentences in conversational speech
- Loses the thought in long sentences with clauses
- Exhibits confusion concerning actor and object of verb

Description. Most normal children can produce well-formed sentences by around 3 or 4 years of age, although the sentences may not be completely grammatical. They comprehend higher-level linguistic constructions sometime between the ages of 5 and 10. Language-disabled students often find it difficult to process sentences that compress the syntactic structure by omitting prepositions. When sentence forms deviate markedly from simple subject, verb, and object phrases, the language-impaired student may guess at the meaning, or deep structure, without trying to decode the relationships among the words, or surface structure, of the sentence. This is particularly true of oral sentences, which must be decoded immediately since the discourse is continuing and the listener cannot stop to study an unusual syntactic structure. The language-disabled student may keep listening, hoping for cues that will indicate the message content in some comprehensible way. If the cues are not present, the student may really have little understanding of information presented in long, complex sentences containing phrases, clauses and unfamiliar verb forms.

Causation. It seems that one of the basic deficiencies in the linguistically handicapped student is the inability to organize verbal information. This student ordinarily is slow in learning to produce a complete simple sentence and may continue to use disjointed phrases when attempting to impart information that must be clarified, expanded, or qualified. Others in his daily environment may use only simple sentence constructions; therefore, the student may come to school having little prior experience with complex sentences. Since linguistically handicapped students are usually reluctant readers, they seldom have the advantage of seeing unfamiliar sentence structures in print before hearing them in oral discourse.

Implications. Language-disabled students are likely to have difficulty recalling information if they were unsure of the meaning of the sentences when they were originally heard. They may not be able to mentally repeat the message to themselves (reauditorize), a procedure that would strengthen the memory trace, because they cannot reproduce the unfamiliar syntactical structures. The student will probably need a longer time to process complex sentences and frequently will not be able to communicate the information accurately to another person.

CORRECTION Modify these strategies for the student's learning style, needs, and age.
1. *Two to One.* On the chalkboard, write pairs of simple sentences that the students are to combine into 1 sentence. Illustrate several ways of combining 2 simple sentences. Here are a few pairs to get you started:

The white balloon floated away. The balloon had a clown face.

A brown dog ran down the street. The dog had climbed out of its pen.

The girl has flown around the world. She is a flight attendant.
The man has an injured foot. The man kicks the football.
The water came in the door. It came in when it was raining hard.
The telephone rang. I was doing my homework.

2. *Expand.* Show the student how to expand a simple sentence by including when, where, how, and why an action takes place and who or what was involved. Try this simple sentence:

A man gave his dog a bone.

Add when: yesterday
where: downtown
how: by tossing it up in the air
why: the dog was hungry
who: the owner of a store

(Yesterday, downtown, a man who was the owner of a store, gave his dog, who was hungry, a bone by tossing it up in the air.)

3. *Written Expansion.* Give each student a simple sentence; then have them draw slips from boxes marked "when, where, how, why, who, and what." The slips should each have phrases of additional information as indicated on the boxes. Guide students to incorporate the extra information orally into a few sentences. Next, have students rewrite the simple sentence to include the new information, and then read the new sentence to the group to see if it communicates successfully. Here are some examples:

When	*Where*	*How*	*Why*
Last week	in England	slowly	it was old
At 1:00 at	school	with a big smile	so it could grow
After supper	out West	with difficulty	they were angry
Tuesday	in the backyard	like a flash	it was cold
In October	upstairs	without a sound	the bell rang

Sentences	*Who or What*
A boy threw a ball	who was the teacher's child
A girl sat down	who/that got lost in the woods
The cat jumped up	who/that had long hair
The men talked	who/that was famous
Mother cooked a meal	who/that weighed 100 pounds

Help the students add the descriptive phrases, if necessary, so that the resulting sentences will be syntactically correct. Then have students exchange simple sentences and again draw phrases from the boxes to which they have been returned.

4. *Who Did What?* Spend some time diagramming complex sentences on the chalkboard. This may provide a system of organization for the student who has not been able to devise a way of identifying the basic sentence. Then give the student a list of complex sentences with directions to write beside them: A) who or what; B) did (verb); and C) what (direct object, phrase, or predicate nominative). Sentences might look like these:

Kathy plays the violin like an adult. (Kathy plays violin)
Has she told Frank and Barbara the news? (She has told news)
We had ridden on the bus to the game. (We had ridden bus)

46. "WH" QUESTIONS

DETECTION Watch for the student who:
- Uses statements with rising end inflection as questions
- Cannot answer simple "Wh" questions
- Does not question to gain information

Description. One of the principle functions of verbal language is to make it possible to acquire information by questioning. Most normal 3-year-old children can exhaust any adult by their persistent inquiries: What's that? Why? However, this is commonly utilized for labeling and does not require more than the same cue phrase from the child. The use of *who, when, where,* and *how* comes later in the child's language development and appears to be more difficult. Responding to any of the "wh" questions that may be posed by another speaker appears to require more expertise at manipulating concepts and sometimes is late in developing.

Causation. Children whose social environment is unresponsive to their questioning may abandon early attempts to gather information in that way. As parents wearily respond, *"Who* is that?" to the child's "What that?" and then follow with "That is the mailman," they are teaching correct use of the "wh" words. Parents who regard young children as capable of giving information will ask questions about "Who did that?" and "Where are your shoes?" while children not asked to respond to questions will remain unfamiliar with the variety of question forms. Students who are mentally handicapped may not be alert enough to environmental stimuli to pose questions or may not be able to understand the questioning process without specific demonstration and guidance by patient teachers.

Implications. Some young children come to school without the ability to ask what they want to know, while others ask but are perplexed when they must respond to any but the simplest questions. *When* and *where* may be difficult because responses could be as varied as these: *later; after lunch; when Daddy gets home; at Billy's house; in the kitchen;* and *under the table.* Repeated questioning is sometimes necessary to help children focus on the information desired. As students become more proficient in the use of language, their command of questioning and answering increases. Some adolescents suffer a dramatic decline, however, as illustrated by the classic "Where are you going?"/"Out" exchange.

CORRECTION Modify these strategies for the student's learning style, needs, and age.

1. *20 Questions.* Play a version of 20 questions by writing animal names on slips of paper and placing them in a small box. One student draws a slip and answers "wh" (and "how") questions appropriately. The teacher may need to supply or correct some answers. The other students question in turn and may guess the animal's name after receiving an answer. If they are incorrect, they drop out of the game. The student who guesses correctly draws the next slip to continue the game. Some sample questions are:

Where do you sleep?	What are you afraid of?
Where do you live?	What sound do you make?
What do you eat?	What covers your body?
How many legs do you have?	How do you travel?

2. *Ask It All.* Display an action picture and encourage the students to ask questions about it. If they are reluctant, help by asking: Do you know where they are? Do you know what is in the box? Do you know why they are doing that? Then require students to frame the questions.

3. *Interview.* Let older students practice interviewing a person for a magazine story. Another student could be the famous person, previously prepared to answer factual questions correctly and given some freedom to respond to opinion questions. This could be an excellent social studies activity.

4. *Sentence Line-Up.* Read prepared sentences to a group of students standing in a line. Ask the first student whether the sentence tells who, what, when, where, how, or why. If the student answers correctly, she stays at the head of the line or moves up 1 place. If she gives an incorrect answer, she goes to the end of the line. The student at the head of the line at the end of the game wins. Here are some sample sentences:

Mrs. Brown cooked dinner.	The tree fell on the robber.
The boy jumped quickly.	The line was broken by the storm.
The dog ran to the house.	The book was under the table.
After dinner, they all left.	I was tired so I went to sleep.
The kitten mewed loudly.	We played outside.

5. *Reverse Quiz.* Tell students that this is like a TV game show ("Jeopardy") in which you will supply the answers and they will ask the appropriate question. Demonstrate with 2–3 easy examples and then try these answers for starters:

We need fire to keep us warm.
We have telephones so we can talk to people far away.
Ice melts when it gets too warm.
Rocks sink in water since they are heavy.
It seldom snows in Florida because the weather is warm.

6. *Tell Me What.* This exercise is designed to help young children progress from the stage of labeling individual items in a picture to the stage of integrating the items into a meaningful relationship. Display a picture that focuses on 1 activity in which 1 or more persons are engaged. Ask the student, "What is the boy doing?" If the student names items in the picture, say, "Yes, but what is he doing with them?" If the student seems unable to compose an answer, you might suggest, "Is he eating? No? Is he cutting the grass? Yes, that's right, he's cutting the grass. Say, 'He's cutting the grass.'"

7. *Question Time.* Each morning, set aside a brief Question Time. Ask a simple question of each student and then help her to pose a question to you (a helper may need to whisper in her ear). Sample questions could be:

How old are you?	How did you get to school?
Where is your coat?	What is your sister's name?
Where do you live?	What did you have for breakfast?
Who is your friend?	What is your phone number?

47. SEQUENCING

DETECTION Watch for the student who displays:

- Inability to repeat a short sentence exactly
- Transpositions of sounds or words
- Use of unusual word order or phrases instead of sentences
- Poor rote memory

Description. Sequencing includes the ability to be aware of the various components of a stimulus as well as the ability to reproduce those components in the same order. Stimuli are received in a temporal order and/or a spatial order. Human speech is based on the ability to perceive, remember, and reproduce sounds in a specific order. Reading and writing are based on the ability to recognize printed symbols and their associated sounds in a sequential pattern. Some individuals exhibit unusual difficulties in these areas.

Causation. Sequencing of incoming stimuli is an automatic operation of the central nervous system. In some instances, the system appears to be working improperly and the individual does not automatically perceive the stimuli in temporal order. All the sounds of the word may be heard but the person may not have an accurate pattern so that the word can be repeated correctly. Similarly, the pattern for the order of the words in standard sentence frames may not be established to the degree that the student can easily place the words within the frames to express them himself. A deficiency in any of the sensory modalities may weaken the sequencing ability of the nervous system, since the modalities (visual, auditory, tactual, motokinesthetic) interact to reinforce patterns. This is an idiosyncrasy of the nervous system that may not change appreciably as the student matures but specific training can be helpful in managing this problem.

Implications. Sequencing difficulties may complicate language behaviors ranging from the building of words from small units (e.g., sounds or letters) to the construction of the larger thought units that produce orderly discourse. A student may demonstrate great difficulty with spelling, often including the right letters but in jumbled order. His reading efforts may be confounded by reversals (e.g., *saw* for *was*) and tendencies to skip words, phrases, or entire lines. He may say *pasghetti* and *partament* or omit the middle syllables in words like *beautiful.* Speech/language pathologists sometimes note that students have great difficulty in reproducing articulatory positions even immediately following a demonstration. Mathematical calculations may be incorrect because of transposed digits, and phone numbers may be misdialed for the same reason. When relating events or retelling stories, the student may reproduce the information out of order; he may appear to begin in the middle and go both ways as he talks. His conversations may be almost unintelligible as he struggles to convey information using short sentences or phrases, seemingly unable to construct a lengthy or complex sentence.

CORRECTION Modify these strategies for the student's learning style, needs, and age.

1. *See and Say.* Direct students who have difficulty composing a sentence to practice with a given sentence structure. Presented with a picture, the student repeats, "The boy is standing by the car"; subsequent pictures substitute a dog, girl, man, or clown standing by the car and later a tree, house, or bus for the car. Use flannel board figures, allowing the student to point to each while organizing the sentence. Various sentence frames should be presented and taught and practiced in the same manner.

2. *Spell by H-R-W-P.* Use multisensory input whenever possible to assist in sequencing the information. Spelling words should be studied by hearing the word, reading the word, writing the word while naming each letter, and then pronouncing the completed word. Repeat these steps (omitting reading the word) until the student can successfully spell the word. Review words frequently and reinforce learning by requiring the student to use those words in daily lessons.

3. *Listen and Read.* Some students find it helpful to listen to an audiotape of the written material they are reading, while others find it confusing. Reading orally assists in some cases but becomes a distraction if phonic skills are poor. Try these methods of combined visual-auditory stimuli to determine the benefit for each student.

4. *Pack a Bag.* A good game for training sequencing skill is the familiar "I'm going on a trip and I'm going to take . . ." activity. The first student names an article, and the next student repeats the carrier phrase, the article, and adds another. Each student, in turn, must repeat all articles in the correct sequence. Vary the game by changing the focus of the introductory sentence as in these:

     For my birthday I hope I get . . .
     I went to the zoo and I saw . . .
     I went to the store and I bought . . .

5. *First to Last.* Guide the student to give directions for accomplishing familiar tasks, such as making a peanut butter and jelly sandwich or going from the classroom to the cafeteria. Then have her give instructions for completing a particular class assignment. Discuss assistive strategies, such as writing or thinking key terms.

6. *Sequence Medley.* Place a series of small pictures before the student briefly, remove and shuffle them, and then ask the student to replace them in the same order. Begin with a single category of 3 pictures and gradually increase the number of pictures and the lexical categories. Help the student to remember the sequence by composing sentences ("The dog ran to the tree by the house and ate an apple.") and saying the sentences aloud as reinforcement. Other suggested activities include singing songs with refrains that repeat sequences (e.g., "Old MacDonald Had a Farm") or giving students slips of paper with the name of a month on each (or letter or day of the week) to place in correct sequence; to track progress, chart completion time.

CHAPTER 14 /
WORD FINDING

48. CIRCUMLOCUTION

DETECTION Watch for the student who:

- Has a limited vocabulary
- Rewords and breaks the rhythm of speech
- Uses incorrect words in sentences

Description. Circumlocution is a speech adaptation used by most of us to some degree. The word itself means "talking around" and describes a speaker's efforts to complete a comment when a specific word is elusive. Young children and students use circumlocutions when they do not know the word that is needed. A child may say, "I went out to the big water where the waves are and the sand" because the word *ocean* is not known. Another student might say, "The lady at the store put my money in that thing, the big machine— she took my money." As people get older, words (especially names) seem to slip away and an introduction to Mrs. Brown could sound like this, "I'd like you to meet—to meet a friend of mine. She lives down the street and has the prettiest flowers in town!" Sometimes even familiar words inexplicably disappear in midsentence and the speaker says, "I went up the—up the, you know, moving stairway in the store" and hope the listener does not notice.

Causation. A very limited vocabulary often results in the use of circumlocutions to complete the communication of ideas. The condition is more acute when a cerebral vascular accident (i.e., stroke) has affected the speech and language areas of the brain. The speaker is sometimes almost unable to produce a connected thought because of the number of circumlocutions employed. In addition, the speaker finds words capriciously substituting themselves in conversational speech. Sometimes the words are associated in some way, while at other times, they merely sound alike, but they are not the words the speaker intends to say at all! It appears that the nerve synapses that permit the retrieval of words are working imperfectly and are presenting words that are recognizably related but incorrect. The poststroke speaker might say, "I wanted to make a—you know, with the two breads; so I got the spoon—no— the one with the sharp edge and put on the putter."

Implications. The student who exhibits frequent circumlocutions needs help in vocabulary building so that communication and cognition can keep pace with experiential learning. The observed speech behavior may be an indication of a learning disability in the area of language with specific problems of word recall and organization of concepts. Attention should be directed toward strengthening the stimuli, diminishing the distractions, focusing the student's attention, and providing external motivation.

CORRECTION Modify these strategies for the student's learning style, needs, and age.

1. *In the Room.* Attempt to increase word retrieval efficiency by timed naming exercises. Ask the student to name as many items as possible during 1 minute in these areas: kitchen, living room, school library. After time has elapsed, discuss other items that might have been included. At the next session, repeat the exercise with a 2-minute time period.

2. *Name It.* Obtain picture dictionaries or some of the picture word books now available in bookstores and encourage the student to study them. If the student does not read, name the pictures for her; then later have her name the pictures for you. This is a good opportunity to discuss the use of the item, how it looks, how it sounds, how it feels, and who has one. If the student can read, cover the printed words and ask her to name the pictures.

3. *Storytime.* Ask the student to relate a familiar story, noting any circumlocutions. When the story is finished, discuss with the student the word that might have been used at that point and ask her to tell that part of the story again, using the word upon which you have agreed.

4. *Thesaurus.* Obtain a small thesaurus or book of synonyms for each student in the group. Prepare individual lists of words that have been elusive for each student and direct her to choose 3 to record on file cards (1-word heading for each card). Beneath the word, the student is to write 3–5 synonyms from the thesaurus. Add new words to the list as word-finding problems occur and use the thesaurus at regular times to add the words to the file cards.

5. *Category.* This activity provides practice in producing a suitable word under the stress of a time constraint. The students stand in a row or semicircle and the leader stands close enough to bounce a large playground ball to them. Bounce the ball to a student at random and call out the name of a category. The student must respond with the name of a member of that category before the leader counts to 10. Adjust the difficulty of the game to suit the players. Let them practice a few times before counting and remind them that a name can be used only once. Select categories such as these:

Fruits	Clothing	Rivers	Flowers
States	Desserts	Birds	TV Actors
Books	Insects	Cars	Games
Sports	Animals	U.S. Presidents	Foods

6. *Clues.* Students who must rely on circumlocutions may benefit from this practice, which uses associations to lead to the desired word. Read the clues until a student volunteers to give the answer. Although the clues should be ones that are especially helpful to the particular students, these suggestions may help to develop others:

Put it on over your shirt to keep warm; not as heavy as a coat . . .

Something in the classroom; has a door; hang your coats there . . .

You sit in a seat with someone; it goes up, around, and down; it is at the fair . . .

Something sweet for toast; made from red fruit; cooked with sugar . . .

49. WORD ASSOCIATION

DETECTION Watch for the student who:

- Cannot produce the word for a known concept
- Displays distracting behavior when reciting orally
- Makes false starts and rewords often when giving information

Description. Occasionally, some students appear to have unusual difficulty in word retrieval. Their early speech is filled with general words such as *thing, that,* and *something,* and space fillers like *you know, and then,* and *uhm.* They often resort to gestures to clarify their meaning or may abandon the effort and attempt to disguise their failure by distracting behavior (laughing, coughing, changing the subject, etc.). As they get older, they appear to learn concepts normally, judging from their nonverbal behavior. They have little trouble comprehending what is said to them and can choose the correct words for specific usage from a menu of choices. They recognize words correctly but they are deficient in the ability to produce words at will.

Causation. This is a specific language disability that seems to result from some central nervous system disturbance. The conceptual knowledge appears to be intact, since the student will often describe the appearance and use of the object but be unable to produce the word. Older students or adults may be quite specific about the attributes, naming other members of its category and describing how it is different. They may even be able to name the beginning sound and the number of syllables in the word. Another kind of word-finding difficulty is more a semantic than a memory or retrieval problem. The student who is linguistically disorganized may not have a clear concept to recall and must try for the best fit from several impressions that may not have coalesced adequately.

Implications. The language-disabled student will require a longer time to complete written assignments that require the structuring of responses with his own vocabulary. The student will perform poorly on spontaneous oral recitation. Certain activities that require verbal fluency and proficiency will be quite difficult for the person and career choice should be made with the language disability in mind.

CORRECTION Modify these strategies for the student's learning style, needs, and age.

1. *Learn It.* When teaching new words, use many associations to help the student remember them. Have the student say the word, emphasizing the syllables and accent. Direct the student to write the word, give a definition, and then use it in a sentence. Display a picture that illustrates the word and have the student describe the picture, using the word. Review the same words each day for a week and then have the student write each one on a 3" x 5" card to be kept in a permanent personal file. If needed, have students find magazine or catalog pictures to illustrate each word and paste the pictures on the backs of the word cards.

2. *File It.* Direct or guide the students to alphabetize their cards. Have students insert in the file behind each card or add to the cards themselves such associative information as a picture, synonyms, the name of the story from which it came, or the subject area (science, social studies, math).
3. *File Drill.* Have daily 5-minute file drills during which the teacher says a word and the students compete to be the first to find it in the file. A member of the opposite team must then name an object associated with the word and tell something about it. This can be a team contest with a running score kept for 6 weeks.
4. *Storytell.* Ask the student to tell a story about a given picture, allowing 3 minutes for preparation before the oral presentation. When the exercise is repeated, reduce preparation time to 2 minutes, then 1 minute, finally asking the student to speak extemporaneously about the picture. Urge the student to tell a real story about what is happening. Be sure the pictures contain enough action to suggest an interesting story.
5. *Pizza Pie.* Prepare a large cardboard round, such as is used to hold a pizza by marking in 8 pie-slice wedges. Print a category name on a gummed label and affix 1 to each wedge. Make a spinner from cardboard and fasten to the center of the cardboard round with a metal paper fastener. Discuss the categories with students and guide them to name at least 3 items that exemplify each. Then have them spin and name a member of the listed category on which the spinner stops. Categories can be subdivided for more capable students: Food (fruit, vegetables, meat); Animals (mammals, fish, insects); Plants (flowers, trees, field crops); or Cities (in our state, out of our state, outside the country).
6. *Analogies.* Help students to see relationships by analogies. Demonstrate the concept by using actual objects or pictures, such as a dog/puppy and cat/kitten. Discuss the relationships and then present the analogy format. Guide students to complete statements such as these:

> Gloves are to hands as shoes are to _____ (feet)
> Hair is to dogs as feathers are to _____ (birds)
> Hands are to people as paws are to _____ (cats)
> Gas is to cars as food is to _____ (people)
> Kittens are to cats as cubs are to _____ (bears)
> Eggs are to chickens as milk is to _____ (cows)
> Knee is to leg as elbow is to _____ (arm)
> Dogs are to bark as ducks are to _____ (quack)
> Hall is to school as street is to _____ (city)

7. *Closure.* Reinforce previously learned phrases by asking the student to complete sentences such as these:

> I will write a note if I can find paper and a _____.
> Wait till I put on my shoes and _____.
> I set the table with the forks, knives, and _____.
> At the party we ate ice cream and _____
> The girl was wearing a skirt and _____.
> May I have some bread and _____?
> On Thanksgiving, we eat _____.

50. CONCEPTUAL CATEGORIZATION

DETECTION Watch for these behaviors:

- Inability to spontaneously group into obvious categories
- Poor or absent use of synonyms in speech and written work
- Inability to sort in more than one way

Description. This ability involves recognizing similar attributes of objects and people that are nonidentical. This ability is developmental in nature and is also related to level of intelligence.

Causation. The language-disordered youngster who has difficulty understanding and making abstractions will also likely experience problems in categorizing. Limited vocabulary may stem from the inability to recognize commonalities in objects, words, expressions, and feelings.

Implications. The student who is unable to create a conceptual scheme for categorization will likely experience failure or great difficulty in academic subjects, including reading, composition, social studies, science, economics, and problem solving in general. He may have difficulty adapting to unfamiliar social situations because of his inability to determine similarities to previous experiences.

CORRECTION Modify these strategies for the student's learning style, needs, and age.

1. *Shape, Size, Color Group.* Arrange 3 blue squares of graduated sizes and 3 red circles of graduated sizes on the table. Demonstrate physically and verbally that the objects can be grouped by color or by size. Mix the shapes and tell the student to group them in 2 different ways. Reinforce correct categorizations. Reteach if the performance was incorrect. Add 3 yellow triangles of graduated sizes to the array. If the child has been successful with the reds and blues, tell him to categorize the objects 3 ways. If he has not been successful, demonstrate then have him imitate. Continue adding different shapes and colors.

2. *Exploring Categories.* Present pictures of a giraffe and a dog. Explore with the child similar attributes of the animals. Write down each attribute. Categorize as "animals." Add a picture of a tiger. Check each attribute listed for the other 2 animals to test whether a tiger is an animal. Add pictures of several animals and follow the same procedure. When the child has mastered this task, present a picture of a tree. Go through the exercise so that the child can determine that the tree does not have the same attributes as the animals and therefore is not an animal. Repeat this exercise with numerous categories of concrete objects, such as flowers, foods, money, balls, toys, candy, and anything else the child finds motivating.

3. *Abstract Categorization.* When the child has sufficiently mastered categorization of concrete objects, introduce more abstract concepts (feelings, democratic ideals, entrepreneurship) and more difficult to categorize words.

4. *Spider Webbing.* Teach the student how to create a semantic map. Begin with concrete objects for ease of learning. Write the word *dog* in the center of a circle. Draw spokes (as on a bicycle or a spider web) radiating from the center. Each spoke should end in a circle in which is written 1 attribute of the central word. (Sample attributes for *dog* may include *animal, four-legged, pet, mammal.*) On another sheet of paper, write the word *giraffe* and circle it. Repeat the activity of drawing spokes with attributes encircled. Compare the 2 maps or webs. If there is at least 1 similar attribute, then the 2 can be associated. Add other animals for practice. Create webs with fruit, sports, people, and so on.

5. *Synonym Selection.* Prepare a sentence in which a noun is highlighted. Repeat the sentence, omitting the highlighted noun and provide a selection of synonyms from which 1 choice is appropriate.

   Sample sentences:

   a. The report of the experiment was well written.
   The _____ of the experiment was well written.
   (account, statement, word)

   b. Her credit limit was raised to $7,500.
   Her credit _____ was raised to $7,500.
   (deadline, restriction, termination)

   c. His comments caused doubt to be planted in her mind.
   His comments caused _____ to be planted in her mind.
   (question, skepticism, suspicion)

   d. She selected a thick novel to read while on vacation.
   She selected a thick _____ to read while on vacation.
   (fiction, book, story)

   Create sentences highlighting other parts of speech (verbs, adjectives, adverbs).

6. *Thesaurus Tic-Tac-Toe.* This can be a game between 2 students or a solitary activity. Prepare a Tic-Tac-Toe grid with 1 word printed in the center box. In order to score an X, the student must provide a noun synonym. In order to score an O, the student must provide a verb synonym.

7. *Odd Man Out.* Prepare groups of words in which 3 are related and 1 is not. The student should identify which one doesn't belong. Have the student verbalize in which way 3 are alike and 1 is different.

   Sample series:

   ball, bat, net, racquet
   belt, shirt, tie, whistle
   computer, dress, pencil, typewriter
   blue, green, red, white
   banana, corn, pear, strawberry
   cheese, egg, fish, oatmeal
   automobile, bicycle, scooter, skate board
   staple, zipper, button, velcro
   adjective, noun, object, verb

CHAPTER 15 /
SPECIAL LANGUAGE PROBLEMS

51. ECHOLALIA

DETECTION This may be the problem of a student who:
- Repeats others' comments verbatim
- Repeats statements made earlier by others
- Imitates inflections as well as words
- Does not refer to himself as "I" or "me"
- Began talking later than expected

Description. Echolalia is a marker of a normal stage of language development in the young child. It usually occurs after a few functional words have been produced and the child has tuned in to speech as an interesting and desirable activity. The child's articulation is fairly consistent although often imprecise and there appears to be satisfaction in trying new sound combinations. It seems that vocal ability has progressed beyond vocabulary and syntactical skills, so the young child is willing to practice on others' words and phrases. Mothers are sometimes startled by the accurate reproduction of familiar phrases—"Thank you!", "No, no, Baby," "I love you," and "Baby want to go bye-bye"—complete with original inflectional pattern. This is a fleeting stage with most children, who soon develop enough vocabulary and rudimentary understanding of syntactical rules to string together their own words. There are some individuals, however, who appear to get stuck at this stage. These children continue to echo what is said to them and seldom produce any words spontaneously.

Causation. It is possible that some central nervous system disorder has affected the language decoding and encoding functions of the echolalic child. These students usually do not produce first words at the expected time, but after much urging from parents, begin to repeat a few single words. They usually repeat "Mama" in what appears to be a normal fashion but they may use it in the presence of any adult. They may develop a strong interest in an object or an activity that can be used to elicit vocalization. Mothers will ask, "Do you want a cookie?" and the echolalic child will respond, "You want a cookie?" Although the child's desire for the cookie may be demonstrated by his gestures, he cannot state that desire. It is apparent that the child's reception of speech is adequate and his phonological system is working well because the words are usually clear. There is, however, a failure of comprehension. The child's words are usually a devitalized rendition of the original speaker's inflections, a hollow parroting of words without expression in the eyes or face. The child is performing like a tape recorder and sometimes indeed whole sentences are produced that seem to be spontaneous but can be recognized as delayed playback of previously heard speech.

Implications. Parents, teachers, and speech pathologists must curb their inclination to ask the child to repeat words in an effort to build vocabulary. This, after all, is what the child already does too well. The echolalic student needs repeated exposure to simple activities that involve the natural use of language. Sentences should be short and simple in structure, with the vocabulary related to the immediate objects and activities.

CORRECTION Modify these strategies for the student's learning style, needs, and age.

1. *Say This.* When the student repeats a greeting verbatim, as in "Hello, John," say, "No, John, you say—'Hello, Aunt Jane,'" dividing the words of your direction from what he is to say with a pause. In the same way, teach him to say, "I'm fine" in response to the query "How are you?"

2. Guess What? When the student wants something but does not know how to express the desire, try to determine what he wants by questioning him: "Do you want a pencil? Do you want paper?" You may have to offer various items until the student indicates that you have guessed correctly. At that point, provide the appropriate sentence by saying, "You say—'I want a pencil.' Now you try it." Do not withhold the item from the frustrated student, but repeat the sentence and praise any partial response.

3. *Talk about It.* When sharing the same visual experience (e.g., looking at a book or watching a videotape), verbalize simple observations in short sentences but do not ask the student to repeat. You might say, "Look, Adam, there's a horse. It's a big brown horse. It is standing by the gate." If you repeat the experience, do not use the same words in your comments. You could say, "I see the horse. The horse is by the gate. It is big and brown." All through the day, adults can attempt to verbalize the student's experiences. Try to imagine his thoughts as he observes, manipulates objects, hears environmental sounds, eats, and plays. If he begins to repeat your sentences, do not praise him but accept the effort and expand the thought. If you say, "The picture is pretty" and he repeats your words, say,"Yes, the sun is shining."

4. *No Parroting.* Echolalic students often memorize commercials heard on TV or radio and can deliver them with amazing accuracy. Resist the temptation to have the student perform this verbal trick for others. Do not reinforce this behavior but try to provide sentences with communicative value to the student. For example, "My name is Donald Allen. My parents are Jerry and Joyce Allen. We live at 415 Lakeshore Drive, Marshall, Illinois. Our telephone number is 373–2340."

5. *Say Another Way.* Use pictures of familiar or high-interest objects in the attempt to develop a spontaneous vocabulary. Be careful to use a different phrase each time the picture is presented. For instance, the same picture might be presented in these ways:

This is a blue bird.	The bird is sitting on the branch.
Do you see the bird's wings?	Where are the bird's eyes?

Encourage the student to respond when the picture is presented, rewarding him with some small token if he names the subject. If he does not, you make a short statement about the picture and continue to the next.

52.   DELAYED LANGUAGE

DETECTION Watch for the student who:

- Does not begin to talk at the normal age
- Does not learn new words easily
- Uses only a few words or phrases for communication

Description. *Delayed language* is a general term to describe the failure of a child to communicate adequately through the spoken word. Speech is the oral expression of language and it is not an inborn but a learned skill. However, most normal children have acquired a basic understanding of the language system and intelligible, functional speech by the age of 4 or 5 without it ever having been formally taught. Unfortunately, some children do not begin to talk at the expected age of 12 to 18 months, causing their parents increasing concern as time passes and speech still does not appear. More and more children, particularly those between the ages of 2 and 5, are being referred for professional evaluation because their speech production is limited. *Delayed language* ordinarily is used to describe language that follows the normal developmental pattern but progresses at a slower rate. A noticeable deviation from the normal pattern is more often called a *language disorder.*

Causation. The term *delayed language* refers only to the observed behavior of children and is not a diagnostic pronouncement. There are many possible causes for this behavior and its manifestation is varied in kind and degree. Delayed language may result from organic dysfunction, such as hearing or visual impairment, but often a specific cause cannot be identified. Certain problems may be noted in the language-delayed child, such as central nervous system impairment, mental retardation, behavior disorder, social or economic deprivation, frail physical health, or immaturity. These conditions may occur separately or in combination and will certainly impede the normal development of language.

Implications. Obviously, different problems will require somewhat different facilitation techniques, but the primary goal is to help the child learn to speak as effectively as possible. The professionals who work with the child should be observant of her responses to a variety of stimuli and varied situations. Information gained in this way may aid in identifying specific problem areas and perhaps modifying them. The ability to communicate with others in one's environment is a critical aspect of human behavior. Intervention by parents, teachers, and speech pathologists can provide experiences, activities, and remedial strategies to encourage and nurture the child's developing speech and language.

CORRECTION Modify these strategies for the student's learning style, needs, and age.

1. *Pick a Pocket.* Prepare a large double (front and back) poster board replica of a coat, tape several library card pockets on it (front and sleeves), and suspend it with a coat hanger between the front and back. Make 3" x 5" cards to fit in the

pockets and paste pictures on one end of the card. The student is to draw a card from a pocket and make a sentence about that picture. Separate pockets can be used for each student and will contain cards with pictures that the student needs to learn. This makes it possible for all students to participate in the same activity while being challenged at their individual levels. Ask another student to repeat the sentence to encourage good speech and good listening.

2. *Card Game.* The same 3" x 5" cards can be used as though playing a card game. Each student in turn draws a card from the stack, shows the card to the other students, names it, and then tells something about it. If the student is successful, the card is kept; if not, it is replaced at the bottom of the card stack. The student with the most cards at the end of the game is the winner.

3. *Categorize.* Use 3" x 5" cards with pictures pasted on one end. Choose 1 from each category: food, clothing, toys, plants, animals, furniture (or things in the house). Place a card on separate lines of a card chart; then have the students draw cards from a stack and place them on the correct category line. It may help to talk about "things we eat, things we wear, things we play with, things that grow, and things that eat and move around."

4. *Bingo.* Prepare 8" x 8" cardboard cards by dividing them with a colored marker into 16 squares. In each square, mount a colored picture of an item whose name you wish to teach. Prepare a card for each student; each card should have the same items but the pictures should not be identical or placed in the same position on the cards. Teach new vocabulary associated with holidays (holiday stickers help in making cards), study units (kitchen items, vacation trips, seasons of the year), or articulation errors. Provide students with markers to place on the pictures, call out words from a master list, and proceed according to the rules of Bingo. The student who calls "Bingo" must name all 4 objects in the completed row.

5. *What's That?* Play audiotapes of environmental sounds and ask the student to choose the correct picture to illustrate the source from a selection of 10–15. Use sets available through school supply catalogs or make your own. Suggested sounds for the tape are: doorbell, whistle, dog bark, hammer, typewriter, siren, telephone, running water, piano, car horn, baby cry, people's voices, airplane motor, lawnmower, or clattering dishes.

6. *Pick a Picture.* Prepare groups of pictures (easily assembled from magazines) depicting men, chairs, cars, dogs, babies, hands, or other frequently photographed objects. Display a group of 8–10 and instruct the student to locate the object you describe. For example, you might instruct her to choose the picture of the hand that is greasy, the hand wearing a glove, or the hand with painted fingernails. Be sure that only 1 picture will satisfy the description.

7. *Colors and Shapes.* Give the student a supply of cardboard triangles, circles, and squares in red, blue, green, and yellow. Spread them out on a table and instruct her to move the objects about according to directions such as these: Put the red circle on the blue square; put 2 yellow squares on a green triangle; put 3 green circles over the yellow triangle; or put a blue square under a green circle.

53. PROSODIC FEATURES

DETECTION Watch for one or more of these behaviors in a school-aged child:

- Inappropriate response to variations of pitch, duration, loudness, and rhythm
- Inappropriate use of variations of pitch, duration, loudness, and rhythm

Description. Prosody may be described as the voicing patterns of the utterance with respect to loudness, pitch, duration, and rhythm. The combinations of loudness, pitch, duration, and rhythm combine with verbal utterances to express such emotions as love, happiness, shame, fear, sarcasm, anger, surprise, and the like. Understanding and use of prosodic features contribute to the overall communication between speaker and listener. These voicing patterns may confirm or contradict the spoken message. Consider the answer to this question: "Will you please do 3,492 push-ups?" The verbal response is, "Oh, sure." Read silently with no evident prosodic features, the response seems to affirm that the responder is willing to perform the requested physical task. The spoken response with prosodic features noted, however, gives a more accurate indication of the intended meaning of the response. "Oh" (emphasized) (pause of one second), "Sure" (emphasized) (sarcastic tone of voice) would indicate that the responder considers the request to be ridiculous in nature. Contrast that response with "Oh" (no emphasis) (pronounced lightly and quickly) (slight pause) "Sure" (emphasized) (slightly lengthened duration) (slightly higher pitch of initial vowel sound) which would indicate that the responder would be delighted to comply with the request. Perhaps the classic example of use of prosody is found in the following sentence, punctuated to indicate the prosodic features. Compare "What's that in the road ahead?" with "What's that in the road? A head?" The written word in dialogue contains no prosodic features. Authors use adjectives, adverbs, and punctuation to convey meaning beyond that which is written so that the reader may obtain the full richness of the communication. Playwrights use staging directions to assure that their words are spoken with the intended meaning.

Causation. Inability to *understand* prosodic features of language may have its origin in low intellectual functioning, impaired hearing, impaired vision, receptive language dysfunction, and/or impaired affective functioning. Inability to *use* prosodic features of language may originate from the same sources as the inability to understand prosody.

Implications. The student who does not understand meaning conveyed by use of prosodic features in oral communication invariably will have difficulty in academic pursuits and in interpersonal relationships. Much of the learning that takes place in the classroom is dependent upon a combination of the written and spoken word. When these forms of communication are not fully understood or are misunderstood by the student, faulty learning or failure to learn occurs. In interpersonal relationships, the major form of communication is the spoken word. The individual who interprets vocal utterances without regard for the confirmation or contradiction that prosodic features contribute to the utterance will experience social difficulties. Similarly, the student who does not use prosodic features in oral communication in the classroom or in social situations is not likely to experience much success in either arena. Frustration may result, which may impair affective functioning.

CORRECTION Modify these strategies for the student's age, needs, and learning style.

1. *Deciphering Video Puzzles.* Videotape short appropriate action scenes from television situation comedies using VCR equipment. Audiotape 2 versions of short phrases using different prosodic features in each of the phrases that will result in different meanings. Play enough of 1 scene for the student to understand the gist of the activity. (It may be helpful to prepare the student by telling him what he is going to see.) When the target scene is shown, press the mute button so there is no sound. Play the 2 versions of the audiotape and ask the student to select the appropriate version. If the student makes the appropriate selection, praise him for his decision and point out why his decision was appropriate. Also discuss why the other selection would have been inappropriate. If the student makes an inappropriate selection, explain why the other selection is more desirable. Replay the scene so that the student may make the appropriate selection.
   Sample phrases for recording:

Oh, dear.	That made me so happy.
Good move.	I love you, too.
What is that?	You finished your homework?

2. *Low-Tech Video Puzzles.* If video and audio equipment are unavailable or undesirable, the above activity can be carried out with still pictures and live voice. Pictures may be selected from photographs, postcards, greeting cards, magazines, coloring books, comic books, or any appropriate commercial source. The teacher should practice oral delivery of the phrases using differing intensity, pitch, duration, and rhythm before conducting the activity.

3. *The Play's the Thing.* Select an interesting but simple scene from a play. Discuss the scene with the class, noting the actions and the feelings of the characters. Appoint some students to portray the characters. Discuss stage directions for delivery of lines. Demonstrate how use of different prosodic features can change the intent of the playwright.

54. KINESICS

DETECTION Watch for one or more of these behaviors in a school-aged student:

- Inappropriate response or failure to respond to kinesics
- Inappropriate or absent use of kinesics

Description. Kinesics may be described as nonlinguistic cues that facilitate communication, such as gestures, facial expressions, head and body movements, and posture. Kinesics may accompany or take the place of verbal communication. Gestures are arbitrary movements that are interpreted on the basis of convention and may be culture specific (i.e., a gesture that is commonly known and used in American culture may convey an altogether different message in another culture). Facial expressions and head and body movements enhance the communicative process but may also replace verbal communication. Posture, or position of the body, also serves to contribute to communication either by confirming, contradicting, or neutralizing verbal messages.

Causation. A student's inability to understand kinesics may result from any number of causes: low intellectual functioning, impaired hearing, impaired vision, receptive language dysfunction, and/or impaired psychological functioning. The inability to use kinesics appropriately may have its origin in low or diminished intelligence, impaired motor functioning, expressive language dysfunction, impaired vision, and/or impaired affective functioning.

Implications. Lack of ability to understand and use gestures, facial expressions, and body posture will undoubtedly have an adverse effect on the student's facility to communicate both when receiving and sending messages. This, in turn, is likely to negatively affect academic achievement and interpersonal relationships with family and peer groups. The student who cannot appropriately interpret the teacher's folded arms, stiff upper body, and tapping foot may be unaware that his behavior is being judged unacceptable by that teacher. The student who asserts, "Yes, I would like to participate in the game" but sits slumped over with his head hanging down conveys a very different message.

CORRECTION Modify these strategies for the student's age, needs, and learning style.

1. *Matching Moods.* Identify common gestures that should be known to the general public. Arrange to photograph a male model portraying those identified gestures. Repeat this portion of the activity with a female model so that 2 sets of photographs are obtained. Display the photographs of either the male model or the female model to the special student. Using a word bank or strips with the gestures named, the student will match the gesture to the photograph. Alter the number of photographs presented and the abstractness of

the gestures, depending on the severity of the child's deficiency in this task. Gradually increase the complexity of the task until the student can identify all gestures in both male and female models.

2. *Making Gestures.* Videotape the same models from the previous activity performing the gestures. The student will identify the gestures as they are performed by the models.

3. *Lights, Action, Camera!* The teacher will perform the gestures and the student will identify them correctly. Then, the student will perform the gestures in front of a full-length mirror with any needed assistance provided by the teacher. The student will be videotaped doing this activity. Upon playback, the student will identify his own gestures correctly.

4. *Fancy Faces.* Photograph a male model whose facial expressions correspond to an identified list of emotions (e.g., happy, sad, puzzled, stern, disapproving, loving, forgiving, proud, fearful, surprised, angry, relieved, sleepy, stern, etc.). Repeat the photography session with a female model portraying the identical emotions. Display both sets of photographs and instruct the child to match the male and female models on the basis of sameness of expressed emotion.

5. *Pigeonholing.* Prepare labels that correspond to the facial expressions displayed in Activity 4 above. The student will attach the label to the proper facial expression. Adjust the difficulty level of this activity to meet the age and developmental level of the student.

6. *Cartoon Bubbles.* When the student has mastered Activities 4 and 5, present him with Blank Cartoon bubbles. Ask him to create a phrase or sentence that might be said by the person in the photograph. For example, the student might write, "I'm sad because I lost my new pencil" in the bubble to be placed on the sad expression photograph. A variation on this activity may be that the teacher would write the sentence and the student would simply match the sentence to the appropriate facial expression.

7. *Picturing Posture.* Take full-length photographs of the male model displaying selected postures. Do the same with the female model. Poses should include acceptance, pleasure, surprise, rejection, depression, studiousness, elation, displeasure, courtesy, and the like. Progress through the steps of matching male and female postures, labeling the male and female postures, performing the targeted postures, and creating sentences the models might be saying.

8. *Charade Fun.* When the child is sufficiently proficient in identifying and performing appropriate gestures, facial expressions, and postures, organize several students into teams to play Charades. The students should be instructed in the rules of the game. The teacher should carefully select the titles to be performed to arrange for success for the special student. As the child increases his skills, the difficulty level of the titles can be increased.

Suggested titles for the beginner:

Three Little Pigs	*One Fish, Two Fish, Red Fish, Blue Fish*
Mother Goose	*Rudolph, the Red-Nosed Reindeer*
Charlotte's Web	*Snow White and the Seven Dwarfs*

55. PROXEMICS

DETECTION Watch for one or more of these behaviors in a school-aged child:

- Inappropriate or absent response to distance messages
- Inappropriate or absent use of distance messages

Description. *Proxemics* may be described as the distance between speaker and audience or the distance between communicators. In the American culture, a distance between speaker and listener of 0–18 inches is described as intimate. Public distance in American culture is a distance between speaker and listener of 12 feet or more. The type of culture is described here because proxemics are interpreted and used differently in different cultures. It is important to note that proxemics alone do not convey intimacy or aloofness. A political candidate who must be separated from the audience, either for safety reasons or for better viewing by the audience, may transmit a feeling of intimacy by gesture and body posture. Another important factor in proxemics involves the level of the communicators. A parent and child who are engaged in intimate distance communication will send and receive different messages if the parent towers above the child (parent looking downward; child looking upward) versus having the same head height (neither looking upward or downward). In the first case, the parent is displaying dominant behavior and the child is displaying subordinate behavior. In the second case, neither parent nor child is displaying dominant-subordinate behavior. The same scenario may occur in public distances. The school principal who stands during a faculty meeting while the faculty is seated is displaying a sign of dominance; the principal who conducts the meeting from a seated position transmits an aura of collaboration rather than domination. The distance may remain the same but the level of head tilt needed for communication changes.

Causation. Inability to interpret proxemics may result from sensory impairment, intellectual impairment, affective or psychological impairment, and/or receptive language dysfunction. The inability to use proxemics effectively may result from sensory impairment, motor impairment, intellectual impairment, affective or psychological impairment, and/or expressive language impairment.

Implications. As with other nonverbal means of communication, the interpretation and use of proxemics serves to confirm, contradict, enhance, or diminish oral communication. The student who does not understand and use meaning conveyed by proxemics may have difficulty in academic areas and will invariably have difficulty in interpersonal relationships. If this difficulty persists into adulthood, the individual will likely have employment and personal problems.

CORRECTION Modify these activities for the student's age, needs, and learning style.

1. *Distance Photo Study.* Select a photograph in which the main feature is 2 children or 2 adults. Have each student in the class write a 1- or 2-paragraph story about the picture. Choose a few volunteers to read their stories. Direct the discussion to focus on nonverbal aspects of communication including proxemics. Lead the class to discover why they attributed actions, feelings, and the like to the subjects in the photograph. Repeat this activity with other photographs until the special-needs child is successful.

2. *Play-Action Proxemics.* Collect a number of interesting props (wig, purse, baseball cap, whistle, cane, shawl, car keys, tennis racket, jump rope, etc.). Divide the class into small groups. In each group, there will be 2 actors and several observers. The actors will be given a short scenario to perform (coach teaching student how to hit a forehand tennis stroke, young man helping an old lady cross the street, mother teaching child how to start a car, etc.). The actors are to pantomime the scenario and the observers are to note variations in proxemics. After the scenario is concluded, discussion will take place. All students should have the opportunity to perform the roles of actor and observer. The special-needs learner should assume the role of actor only after the teacher rates his comfort level as acceptable.

3. *Barrier Bounce.* Photograph 2 children of the same sex seated in identical chairs facing each other. Photograph the same 2 children seated in the same 2 chairs facing each other with a table between them. Present the 2 photographs and ask which picture depicts "best friends." Guide the student to select the photo without the barrier, if that is not his first selection. If he does select correctly without guidance, discuss how the barrier affects the intimacy of proxemics. If further practice is necessary, stage other similar photographs. The difficulty level of the task may be increased by varying the sex of the subjects, the environment, and the furniture.

4. *Barrier Absent/Barrier Present.* The special-needs child should be instructed in the appropriate use and nonuse of barriers. Barriers should be used to demand distance, to give an air of formality to discussion, and as a defense mechanism for self-protection. The interaction should be barrier free to indicate an air of openness, trust, and intimacy. The teacher should locate or create miniplays in which the dialogues dictate whether the interactions should be barrier absent or barrier present. Doll characters and dollhouse furnishings may be used in the initial stages of learning if the student has difficulty adapting this concept to himself. Once the student has mastered the concept, the miniplays should be enacted by the students.

5. *Hands On/Hands Off.* Many special-needs students need instruction in the appropriate use of touching. Write different situations on 3" x 5" cards in which touching would be appropriate and inappropriate (e.g., approaching a sales clerk in a department store, greeting your grandmother, answering the door when the mail deliverer rings, walking up to your friend at school). Have the student sort the cards into "Hands on" and "Hands off" categories. Guide the student's choices as needed.

REFLECTIONS

1. Words with multiple meanings are stumblings blocks for anyone learning the English language, whether that person is a child or an adult. List five words that have multiple meanings in common usage in your region and give three to five meanings for each. Compose sentences that illustrate each meaning and then compare sentences with a peer.

2. Figurative language is used freely in daily conversation but the expressions may have become so familiar that they are not readily recognized as figures of speech. It is easy to recognize figurative language as it is used in poetry; however, the meaning is sometimes not immediately apparent. Select a poem, note the figures of speech used and explain them to the class.

3. The concepts of space and time are troublesome for all children to learn but especially for the learning-language-disordered student. Observe a kindergarten or first grade-class during the first part of the school day and note what activities the teacher presents to help the children to develop their concepts of space and time. Observe in a special classroom at the same time of day and note whether similar activities are presented.

4. The age and developmental level of a student must be considered when planning corrective activities. Review the suggested strategies for Skill 38, Cause and Effect, and choose one to use with an 8-year-old student and one to use with a high school learning-language-impaired student. Compare your two choices and explain how they differ, how they are similar, and why they were selected for that age.

5. A great deal of teaching can be accomplished within the normal activities of the school day. Think of five different ways to incorporate the teaching of prepositions into opening exercises, lunchtime, art or music period, or playground time. Do this for each of these grade levels: first, fifth, and tenth. Consider if the activities are appropriate for the different ages and if they will be as effective as more traditional drill activities.

6. Semantics, morphology, and syntax together provide the vehicle for verbal language. The opportunity for use and the desire to interact verbally are also of great importance. After briefly reviewing the discussions in this section, explain how these three areas interact in connected discourse and how difficulties in any one of the areas can subtract from efficient communication.

7. Certain morphological forms are used incorrectly so often that students may hear the incorrect usage much more frequently than the correct forms. As you observe in classrooms, note the number of times morphological errors occur as students recite or talk spontaneously. If you were the teacher, how would you counteract this reinforcement of poor grammar? Refer to Skill 42 and Skill 43, especially.

8. Teaching the comprehension and use of complex sentence structure to language-impaired students may require the modification of strategies used with most students. After reading the discussion in Skills 44 and 45, obtain a teacher's manual for a seventh-grade language textbook and see what activities are

suggested for teaching complex sentences. Decide how you could expand or modify those activities to make them more appropriate for a student with specific language difficulties.

9. Questioning is an important avenue to the accumulation of necessary information; yet the art of questioning is seldom directly taught. Choose one of the suggested CORRECTION activities for Skill 46 to use with a group of children as a game. Note the type of difficulties they exhibit and make up a new activity or modify one of the suggested ones to answer the perceived need.

10. The ability to sequence information, receptively and expressively, is of paramount importance in all areas of the language arts. The DETECTION behaviors of Skill 47 are only a partial list of areas of deficiency due to sequencing problems. Talk with several teachers to learn of other areas affected by a sequencing disturbance.

11. Word-finding problems affect most people at times, but discuss the possible basis for the severe disability that affects some persons. Tell how you would attempt to help a second-grader and how you would plan a remediation program for an adult.

12. A language delay and a language disorder differ; review the special language problems in Chapter 15 and then explain these differences.

13. A great deal of human communication is nonverbal. Observe a first-grade classroom and list various kinesic and proxemic messages sent from the teacher and from five students. Repeat your observation in an eighth-grade class and compile another list of messages noted. Be prepared to demonstrate any specific nonverbal message for your peers.

14. Suggestions for recognizing and remediating language disabilities are available from a number of authors. Compare and contrast the information presented in these sources with the material in Chapters 11 through 16:

Bates, E., Bretherton, I., & Snyder, L. (1988). *From first words to grammar.* Cambridge, MA: Cambridge University Press.

Bauer, A. M., & Shea, T. M. (1989). *Teaching exceptional students in your classroom.* Boston: Allyn and Bacon.

Bernstein, D. K., & Tiegerman, E. (Eds.) (1989) *Language and communication disorders in children* (2nd ed.). Columbus, OH: Charles E. Merrill.

Darby, J. K. (Ed.). (1985). *Speech and language evaluation in neurology: Childhood disorders.* Orlando, FL: Grune and Stratton.

Edwards, V. (1986). *Language in a black community.* San Diego, CA: College-Hill Press.

Fey, M. E. (1986). *Language intervention with young children.* San Diego, CA: College-Hill Press.

Gaylord-Ross, R. (1989). *Integration strategies for students with handicaps.* Baltimore: Paul H. Brookes.

Gleason, J. B. (1989) *The development of language* (2nd ed.). Columbus, OH: Charles E. Merrill.

James, S. L. (1988). *Normal language development.* San Diego, CA: College-Hill Press.

Lahey, M. (1988). *Language disorders and language development.* New York: Macmillan.

Lass, N. J., McReynolds, L., Northern, J., & Yoder, D. (Eds.). (1988). *Handbook of speech-language pathology and audiology.* St. Louis, MO: C. V. Mosby.

Lund, N. J., & Duchan, J. F. (1988). *Asssessing children's language in naturalistic contexts* (2nd ed.). Englewood Cliffs, NJ: Prentice-Hall.

Mason, J. M. (Ed.). (1989). *Reading and writing connections.* Boston: Allyn and Bacon.

Mercer, C. D., & Mercer, A. R. (1989). *Teaching students with learning problems* (3rd ed.). Columbus, OH: Charles E. Merrill.

Morris, D. (1977). *Manwatching: A field guide to human behavior.* New York: Harry N. Abrams.

Nippold, M. A. (1988). *Later language development.* San Diego, CA: College-Hill Press.

Owens, R. E., Jr. (1990). *Functional language intervention.* Columbus, OH: Charles E. Merrill.

Owens, R. E., Jr. (1988). *Language development: An introduction* (2nd ed.). Columbus, OH: Charles E. Merrill.

Polloway, E. A., Patton, J. R., Payne, J. S., & Payne, R. A. (1989). *Strategies for teaching learners with special needs* (4th ed.). Columbus, OH: Charles E. Merrill.

Rakes, T. A., & Choate, J. A. (1989). *Language arts: Detecting and correcting special needs.* Boston: Allyn and Bacon.

Reed, V. (1986). *An introduction to children with language disorders.* New York: Macmillan.

Schiefelbusch, R. L. (1986). *Language competence: Assessment and intervention.* San Diego, CA: College-Hill Press.

Schloss, P. J., Schloss, C. N., & Smith, M. A. (1990). *Instructional methods for adolescents with learning and behavior problems.* Boston: Allyn and Bacon.

Schulz, J. B., Carpenter, C. D., & Turnbull, A. P. (1990). *Mainstreaming exceptional students: A guide for classroom teachers* (3rd ed.). Boston: Allyn and Bacon.

Shadden, B. (Ed.) (1988). *Communication behavior and aging: A source for clinicians.* Baltimore, MD: Williams and Wilkins.

Skinner, P. H., & Shelton, R. L. (1985). *Speech, language and hearing, normal processes and disorders* (2nd ed.). New York: Macmillan.

Stark, R. E., & Tallal, P. (1988). *Language, speech and reading disorders in children: Neuropsychological studies.* San Diego, CA: College-Hill Press.

Valletutti, P. J., McKnight-Taylor, M., & Hoffnung, A. S. (1988) *Facilitating communication in young children with handicapping conditions.* San Diego, CA: College-Hill Press.

Wiig, E. H. (1989). *Steps to language competence: Developing metalinguistic strategies.* New York: Psychological Corporation.

Wilcox, M. J., & Campbell, P. H. (1988). *Communication programming from birth to three: A handbook for public school professionals.* San Diego, CA: College-Hill Press.

APPENDIX
INTERNATIONAL PHONETIC ALPHABET

Consonants

Symbol	Key Word	Symbol	Key Word
m	mother	l	led
n	never	r	red
p	pat	ŋ	ring
h	hello	ʃ	shoe
w	wed	tʃ	church
b	bob	ɵ	thumb
k	cot	dʒ	jump
g	got	v	vine
d	dot	s	seal
f	fine	z	zeal
j	yet	ð	them
t	teacher	ʒ	beige
		ʍ	what

Vowels

Symbol	Key Word	Symbol	Key Word
ɨ	Pete	o	pole
I	pit	ɔ	Paul
e	bake	a	pot
ɛ	pet	ɝ	purr
æ	pat	ɚ	doctor
u	pool	ə	alive
ʊ	pull	ʌ	gum

Diphthongs

Symbol	Key Word	Symbol	Key Word
eɪ	pale	ɔɪ	boy
oʊ	door	aɪ	fight
aʊ	wow		

Index

ABOUT THE AUTHORS

PAULETTE J. THOMAS has two decades of experience as an educator, researcher, and administrator. She earned M.S. and Ph.D. degrees from Texas A&M University in Educational Psychology and a B.A. from the University of Southwestern Louisiana in Speech Pathology and Audiology. She is currently Associate Professor of Special Education and Habilitative Services at the University of New Orleans, where she has also served as Assistant Dean of the College of Education. She returned to her present position after serving as Assistant Superintendent for Special Educational Services, Louisiana Department of Education. Her experiences have included providing direct and consultative services to speech, hearing, and language impaired children, youth, and adults. She has functioned as a special education coordinator and an educational diagnostician and has taught undergraduate- and graduate-level courses in speech correction, learning disabilities, study of the gifted, study of exceptional children, and psychoeducational diagnosis. Dr. Thomas is a past president of the Council for Educational Diagnostic Services, a division of the International Council for Exceptional Children. She has published a variety of research studies and presented papers at numerous professional conferences. Dr. Thomas has recently begun a term on the editorial board of *Diagnostique.*

FAIRY F. CARMACK has been an educator of exceptional children for more than 25 years. She received an Ed.D. from Northeast Louisiana University and is certified by the American Speech-Language-Hearing Association as a speech and language pathologist. She provides speech and language therapy to students of all ages in Northeast Louisiana and also is a diagnostician and consultant to residential facilities for mentally retarded adults. She has been the speech and language diagnostician on the multidisciplinary pupil appraisal team of Monroe City Schools and formerly taught academics as well as speech to hearing-impaired youngsters. Dr. Carmack has supervised speech therapy student clinicians, taught diagnostics at the university level, and presented numerous workshops and papers at professional conferences.

READER'S REACTION

Dear Reader:

No one knows better than you the special needs of your students or the exact nature of your classroom problems. Your analysis of the extent to which this book meets *your* special needs will help us to revise this book and assist us to develop other books in the *Detecting and Correcting* series.

Please take a few minutes to respond to the questionnaire on the next page. If you would like to receive a reply to your comments or additional information about the series, indicate this preference in your answer to the last question. Mail the completed form to:

> Joyce S. Choate, Consulting Editor
> *Detecting and Correcting* Series
> c/o Allyn and Bacon
> 160 Gould Street
> Needham Heights, Massachusetts 02194

Thank you for sharing your special needs and professional concerns.

Sincerely,

Joyce S. Choate

Joyce S. Choate

READER'S REACTIONS TO
SPEECH AND LANGUAGE: DETECTING AND CORRECTING SPECIAL NEEDS

Name: _____   Position: _____

Address: _____

_____   Date: _____

1. How have you used this book?

   ___College Text   ___Inservice Training   ___Teaching Resource

   Describe:_____

2. For which purpose(s) do you recommend its use?

3. What do you view as the major strengths of the book?

4. What are its major weaknesses?

5. How could the book be improved?

6. What additional topics should be included in this book?

7. In addition to the topics currently included in the *Detecting and Correcting* series—basic mathematics, classroom behavior, instructional management, language arts, reading, science and health, social studies, and speech and language—what other topics would you recommend?

8. Would you like to receive:

   _____a reply to your comments?

   _____additional information about this series?

Additional Comments:

THANK YOU FOR SHARING YOUR SPECIAL NEEDS AND PROFESSIONAL CONCERNS

**Stepping into Standards
Theme Series**

Down on the Farm

Written by
Kimberly Jordano and Tebra Corcoran

Editor: Teri L. Fisch
Illustrator: Darcy Tom
Cover Illustrator: Kimberly Schamber
Designer: Moonhee Pak
Cover Designer: Moónhee Pak
Art Director: Tom Cochrane
Project Director: Carolea Williams

Table of Contents

Introduction

Due to the often-changing national, state, and district standards, it is often difficult to "squeeze in" fascinating topics for student enrichment on top of meeting required standards and including a balanced program in your classroom curriculum. The *Stepping into Standards Theme Series* will help you incorporate required subjects and skills for your kindergarten and first-grade children while engaging them in a fun theme. Children will participate in a variety of language arts experiences to help them with **phonemic awareness** and **reading** and **writing** skills. They will also have fun with **math activities, hands-on science activities,** and **social studies class projects.**

The creative lessons in *Down on the Farm* provide imaginative, innovative ideas to help you motivate children as you turn your classroom into a farm. The activities will inspire children to explore the farm as well as provide them with opportunities to enhance their knowledge and meet standards.

Invite children to "visit" a farm as they
- participate in phonemic awareness activities that feature theme-related poems and songs
- create mini-books that reinforce guided reading and sight word practice
- contribute to shared and independent reading and writing experiences about farm animals
- practice counting and addition with ants on a picnic
- make observations, collect data, and graph the growth cycle of a plant
- explore farm-grown products
- complete several fun art projects as they turn their room into a farm
- participate in an end-of-the-unit Evening on the Farm to showcase their work

Each resource book in the *Stepping into Standards Theme Series* includes standards information, easy-to-use reproducibles, and a full-color overhead transparency to help you integrate a fun theme into your required curriculum. You will see how easy it can be to incorporate creative activities with academic requirements while children enjoy their adventures on the farm!

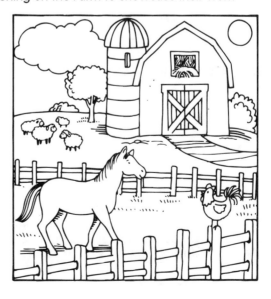

Meeting Standards

Language Arts

	Rhyming on the Farm, page 7	Mr. Farmer, page 7	We're Going to the Zoo, page 12	The Little Pig, page 12	Reading Aloud, page 16	Morning Message, page 17	Pocket Chart Stories, page 18	Sentence Puzzle, page 18	Buzz, Buzz mini-book, page 20	Are They Alive? mini-book, page 24	Professional Piggy Pack, page 28	Down on the Silly Farm, page 28	Horsing Around with Words, page 32	On the Farm, page 32	Piggy Pete, page 34	Farm Fun Number Poem, page 34	On the Silly Farm, page 35	Wishy-Washy Bathtub, page 37	Nibbling Rabbit Mural, page 39	Piggy Tales, page 40
Phonemic Awareness																				
Identify beginning consonant sounds		•	•														•	•	•	
Identify letters		•																•	•	
Identify rhyming words	•															•				
Isolate beginning sounds		•	•	•													•	•	•	
Recognize rhythm and rhyme	•		•													•				
Substitute beginning consonant sounds		•	•														•	•		
Reading																				
Apply phonics concepts									•	•	•	•	•				•			
Apply reading strategies					•	•	•		•	•	•	•				•		•		
Develop awareness of concepts of print						•	•	•	•	•	•		•	•	•	•				
Develop oral language skills	•	•	•			•	•	•	•	•	•	•	•	•	•	•		•		
Identify plot, characters, conflict, and resolution					•															
Improve reading comprehension									•	•	•									
Improve reading fluency									•	•	•	•	•	•	•	•		•		
Improve story comprehension					•				•	•							•	•	•	•
Make predictions					•															
Recognize sight word vocabulary						•	•	•	•	•	•	•		•	•	•	•	•	•	
Track words from left to right						•	•	•	•	•	•	•		•	•	•	•	•	•	•
Writing																				
Apply phonics skills						•			•	•	•		•	•	•	•		•	•	•
Brainstorm and organize ideas														•	•	•	•		•	•
Choose correct punctuation						•									•	•				
Develop focused, detailed writing																			•	•
Follow spelling rules						•			•	•	•		•	•	•	•			•	
Incorporate letter and word spacing						•			•	•	•		•	•	•	•			•	•
Model letter formation						•								•	•			•		
Model sentence structure						•									•					
Practice correct letter formation						•			•	•	•					•	•	•	•	•
Write complete sentences															•				•	•

Meeting Standards

Math
Science
Social Studies

	Mr. Horse's Tasty Treats, page 43	Watermelon Seed Number Book, page 44	Scarecrow Glyph, page 46	Addition Nests, page 48	Ants on a Picnic, page 50	Seasons on the Farm, page 53	Plant a Sunflower Garden, page 53	Who Will Help Me?, page 54	What Did You Grow?, page 56	Evening on the Farm, page 58	Farmer's Hat, page 58	Cooking on the Farm, page 59	Papier-Mâché Rockin' Roosters, page 59	Hayride Hoedown Bulletin Board, page 60	Midnight on the Farm Bulletin Board, page 61
Math															
Add		•		•	•										
Analyze data	•		•												
Count		•	•	•	•										
Count using one-to-one correspondence		•	•		•										
Graph	•														
Subtract		•													
Understand number families						•									
Write numbers correctly	•	•		•	•										
Science															
Collect data							•								
Identify activities that take place in different seasons						•									
Identify parts of a plant									•						
Make observations							•								
Monitor the growth cycle of plants							•								
Understand cyclical changes						•									
Social Studies															
Explore kindness								•							
Practice cooperating with others								•							
Understand why produce is important									•						
Additional Language Arts															
Brainstorm and organize ideas						•									
Develop oral language skills			•	•		•					•				
Follow spelling rules	•	•			•	•	•	•	•	•	•			•	•
Follow step-by-step directions			•						•			•	•	•	
Improve story comprehension						•		•	•			•			
Incorporate letter and word spacing	•	•			•	•	•	•	•	•	•			•	
Practice correct letter formation	•	•				•	•	•	•	•	•			•	•
Write complete sentences					•	•	•								

Instant Learning Environment

This resource includes a full-color overhead transparency of a farm environment that can be used in a variety of ways to enhance the overall theme of the unit and make learning more interactive. Simply place the transparency on an overhead projector, and shine it against a blank wall, white butcher paper, or a white sheet. Then, choose an idea from the list below, or create your own ideas for using this colorful backdrop.

Unit Introduction

Give children clues about the farm unit. For example, say *We are going to study about a place where people and animals live together. Vegetables are grown there. These vegetables are called crops.* Invite children to use the clues to discuss what the unit might be about. Then, display the transparency to give children a quick overview of the environment and an introduction to the unit.

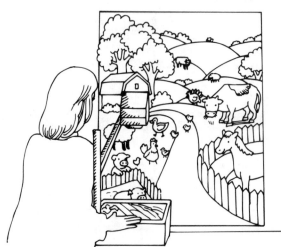

Or, cut out puzzle pieces from an 8½" x 11" (21.5 cm x 28 cm) sheet of paper. Place the puzzle pieces on top of the transparency on the overhead projector so they cover it entirely. Turn on the projector. None of the farm environment will show. Remove one puzzle piece at a time, and describe the uncovered section. Invite children to identify the environment. Then, continue to remove pieces, asking children to predict what they might see next until you have revealed the entire transparency.

Dramatic Play

Use the transparency as a backdrop for children to perform the dramatic play described on page 28. Have children wear a character headband (glue cutouts from the Farm Animals reproducible on page 14 and the Farmer reproducible on page 33 to sentence strips) as they perform.

Farm Spelling

Have children practice spelling farm words at an independent learning center. Project the transparency on a piece of white butcher paper. Have children write the names of the animals and objects in the farm scene (e.g., chicken, barn, tractor). Encourage children to draw and label additional animals.

Phonemic Awareness

ABC
Rhyming on the Farm

MATERIALS

✓ Rhyming Picture Cards
(page 8)
✓ Barn reproducible
(page 9)
✓ tagboard
✓ brown paper bags
✓ art supplies

Copy a class set of the Rhyming Picture Cards on tagboard. Show children a set of picture cards, and have them identify each picture. Give each child a Barn reproducible to color, cut out, and glue to the front of a paper bag. Give each child a set of the cards to cut apart. Invite children to look at their cards and find pairs of pictures that rhyme. As children match each pair, have them say the pairs to a partner or an adult and then put the pair in their bag. To extend the activity, have children practice this activity at home with their family.

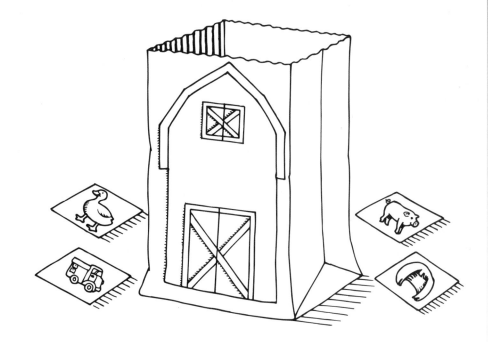

ABC
Mr. Farmer

MATERIALS

✓ "Mr. Farmer" poem
(page 10)
✓ Farm Food Cards
(page 11)
✓ construction paper
✓ tagboard
✓ resealable plastic bags

Copy the poem "Mr. Farmer" on construction paper. Copy a class set of the Farm Food Cards on tagboard, cut them apart, and put each set in a separate plastic bag. Show children a set of food cards, and ask them to identify each food (i.e., carrots, zucchini, lettuce, pumpkin, peas, tomatoes, eggplant, beans). Have them tell what sound each food starts with and what letter it starts with. Give each child a bag of food cards. Read aloud the poem, and have children hold up the appropriate card at the end of each stanza. To extend the activity, use the additional food cards to make up other stanzas.

Rhyming Picture Cards

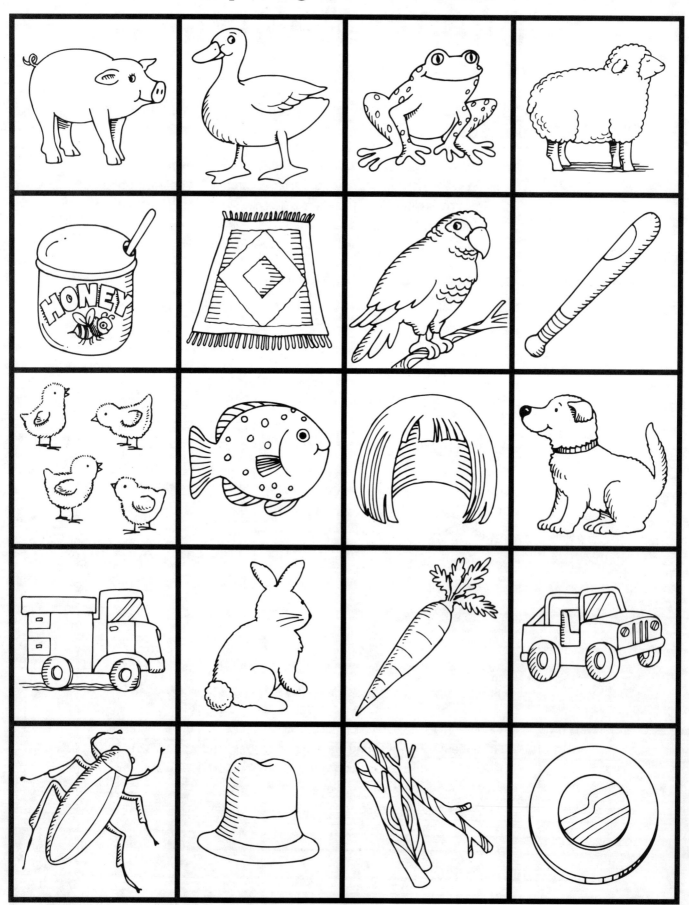

Barn

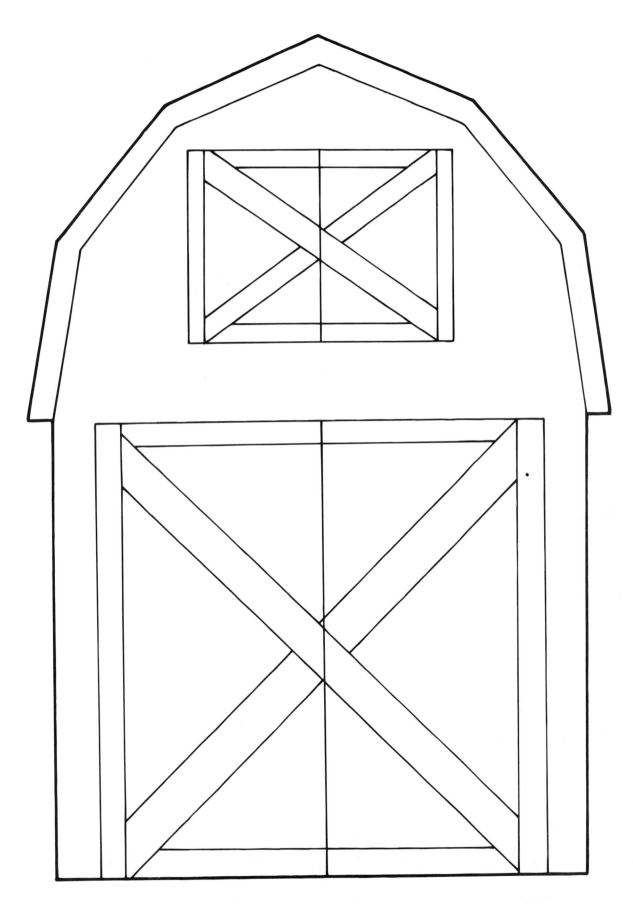

Mr. Farmer

(read to the tune of "Frere Jacques")

Mr. Farmer, Mr. Farmer,
Please tell me, please tell me.
What's growing in your garden?
What's growing in your garden?
It starts with /k/. It starts with **C.**

Mr. Farmer, Mr. Farmer,
Please tell me, please tell me.
What's growing in your garden?
What's growing in your garden?
It starts with /p/. It starts with **P.**

Mr. Farmer, Mr. Farmer,
Please tell me, please tell me.
What's growing in your garden?
What's growing in your garden?
It starts with /e/. It starts with **E.**

Mr. Farmer, Mr. Farmer,
Please tell me, please tell me.
What's growing in your garden?
What's growing in your garden?
It starts with /t/. It starts with **T.**

Mr. Farmer, Mr. Farmer,
Please tell me, please tell me.
What's growing in your garden?
What's growing in your garden?
It starts with /z/. It starts with **Z.**

Mr. Farmer, Mr. Farmer,
Please tell me, please tell me.
What's growing in your garden?
What's growing in your garden?
It starts with /l/. It starts with **L.**

Farm Food Cards

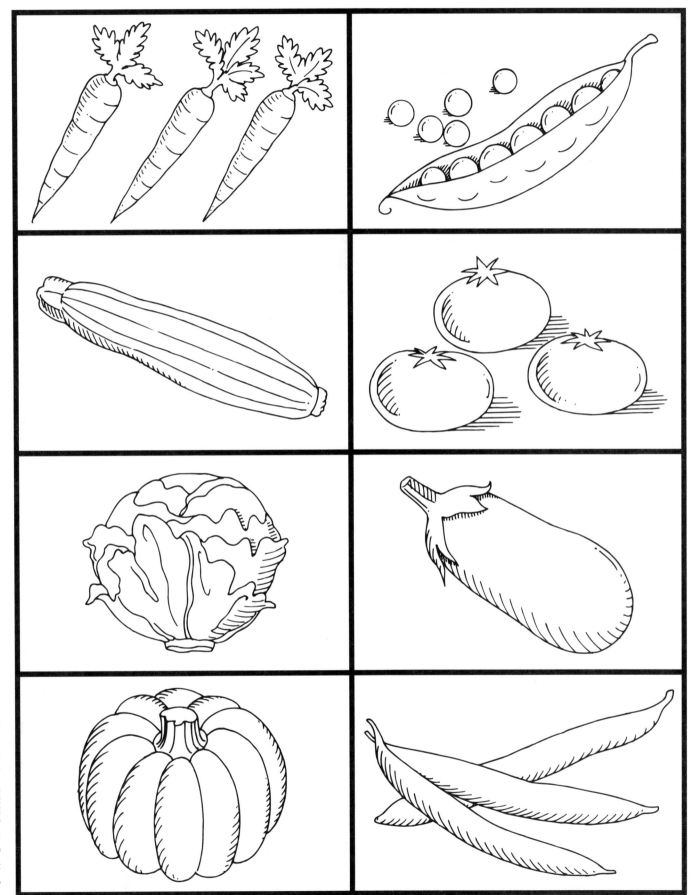

We're Going to the Farm

M A T E R I A L S

✓ "We're Going to the Farm" song (page 13)
✓ Farm Animals reproducible (page 14)
✓ red construction paper
✓ craft sticks
✓ art supplies

Copy the song "We're Going to the Farm" on red construction paper. Give each child a Farm Animals reproducible. Have children color the cow, lamb, horse, and pig, cut them out, and glue them on separate craft sticks to make puppets. Sing the song. Have children use the sound of the first letter of the name of one of their animals to replace the first letter of each word of *hi-ho the derry-o*. For example, when children sing the line about the lamb, they say *li-lo the lerry-o*. Have children hold up the appropriate farm animal puppet for each line. To extend the activity, invite children to make up additional verses about the other animals on the Farm Animals reproducible.

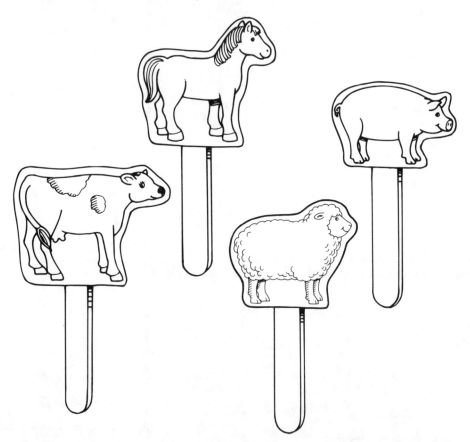

The Little Pig

M A T E R I A L S

✓ "The Little Pig" song (page 15)
✓ pink construction paper
✓ pig stuffed animal

Copy the song "The Little Pig" on pink construction paper. Sing the song. Replace each bolded name with a child's name, and toss a pig stuffed animal to him or her. Replace the first sound of the child's name with /p/. Continue singing the song until you have said each child's name. To extend the activity, use a different stuffed animal and the beginning sound of that animal as you sing the song. For example, if you use a horse, you will say *Hickety, hackety, hee, / A horse flew over me. / Hickety, hackety, hoo, / The horse flew over to you!* Invite children to sing the song with you and change the beginning sound accordingly.

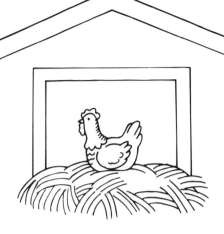

We're Going to the Farm

(sing to the tune of "The Farmer in the Dell")

We're going to the farm. We're going to the farm.
Fi-fo the ferry-o, it's time to see the farm!

I hope we see a cow. I hope we see a cow.
Ci-co the cerry-o, I hope we see a cow!

I hope we see a lamb. I hope we see a lamb.
Li-lo the lerry-o, I hope we see a lamb!

I hope we see a horse. I hope we see a horse.
Hi-ho the herry-o, I hope we see a horse!

I hope we see a pig. I hope we see a pig.
Pi-po the perry-o, I hope we see a pig!

I think it's time to go. I think it's time to go.
Gi-go the gerry-o, I think it's time to go!

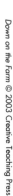

Farm Animals

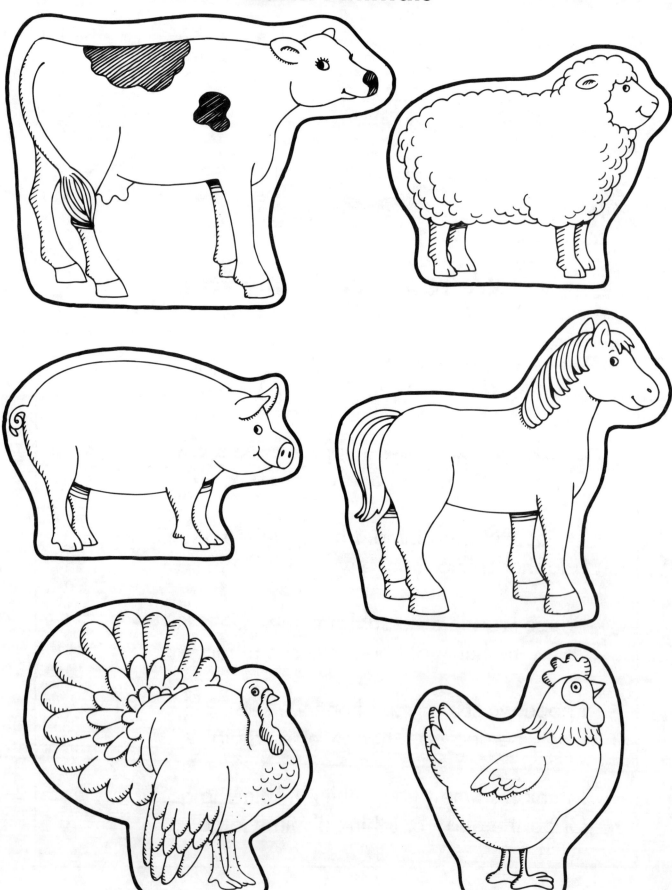

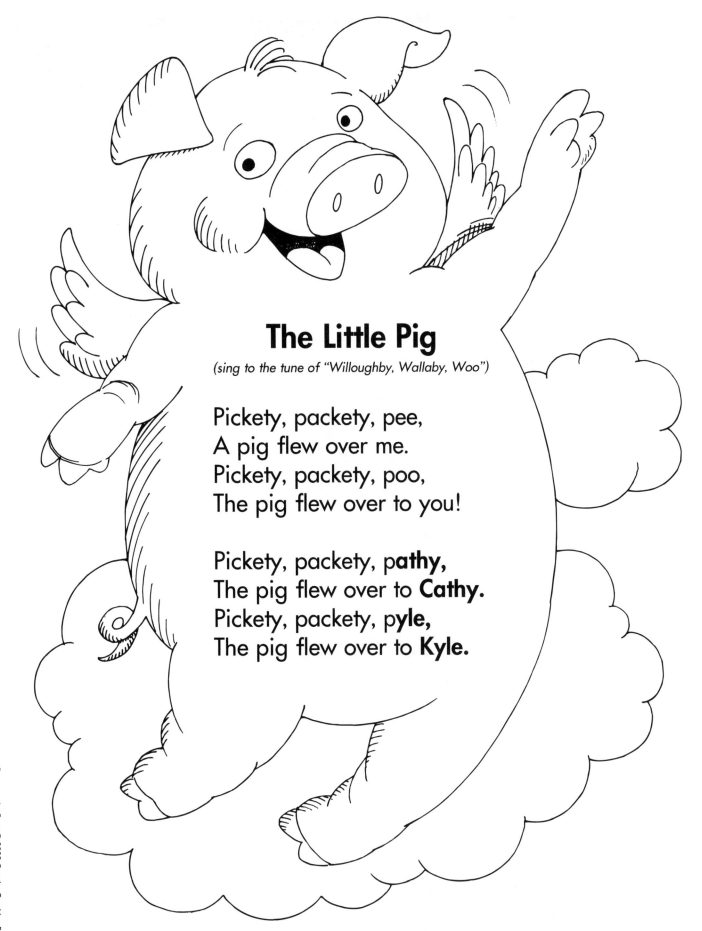

The Little Pig

(sing to the tune of "Willoughby, Wallaby, Woo")

Pickety, packety, pee,
A pig flew over me.
Pickety, packety, poo,
The pig flew over to you!

Pickety, packety, p**athy**,
The pig flew over to **Cathy**.
Pickety, packety, p**yle**,
The pig flew over to **Kyle**.

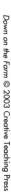

Modeled Reading

Introduce the farm to your class by reading aloud books from the following literature list or others with similar content. Invite children to look at the book cover and pictures and discuss what they see. Ask them to predict what the book will be about and to point out animals, plants, and details that relate to the farm.

Literature List

Barn Dance by Bill Martin Jr. and John Archambault (Henry Holt and Company)

Barnyard Banter by Denise Fleming (Owlet)

Buzz Said the Bee by Wendy Cheyette Lewison (Scholastic)

Career Day by Anne Rockwell (HarperCollins)

The Chick and the Duckling by Mirra Ginsburg (Aladdin)

Chickens Aren't the Only Ones by Ruth Heller (Price Stern Sloan)

Cock-A-Doodle-Moo! by Bernard Most (Harcourt)

The Cow That Went Oink by Bernard Most (Harcourt)

The Easter Egg Farm by Mary Jane Auch (Holiday House)

Eating the Alphabet: Fruits and Vegetables from A to Z by Lois Ehlert (Voyager Books)

A Field of Sunflowers by Neil Johnson (Cartwheel Books®)

Growing Vegetable Soup by Lois Ehlert (Voyager Books)

Harvey Potter's Balloon Farm by Jerdine Nolen and Mark Buehner (Mulberry Books)

I Like Me! by Nancy Carlson (Viking)

I Went Walking by Sue Williams (Voyager Books)

In the Garden by David M. Schwartz (Creative Teaching Press)

Inside a Barn in the Country: A Rebus Read-Along Story by Alyssa Satin Capucilli (Scholastic)

Jobs People Do by Christopher Maynard (DK Publishing)

The Little Duck by Judy Dunn (Random House)

The Little Red Hen by Paul Galdone (Houghton Mifflin)

The Midnight Farm by Reeve Lindbergh (Dutton)

Mrs. Wishy-Washy by Joy Cowley (Philomel)

My First Farm Board Book (DK Publishing)

The New Baby Calf by Edith Newlin Chase (Scholastic)

One Cow Moo Moo! by David Bennett (Henry Holt and Company)

Piggy Pie! by Margie Palatini (Houghton Mifflin)

Pigs in the Mud in the Middle of the Rud by Lynn Plourde (Scholastic)

The Reason for a Flower by Ruth Heller (Price Stern Sloan)

The Red Barn by Margaret Wise Brown (HarperFestival)

The Seasons of Arnold's Apple Tree by Gail Gibbons (Voyager Books)

The Tale of Peter Rabbit by Beatrix Potter (Frederick Warne)

Time for Bed by Mem Fox (Red Wagon Press)

Shared Reading

Morning Message

✓ chart paper or dry erase board
✓ markers or dry erase markers
✓ Wikki Stix® (optional)
✓ reading stick

Turn your morning message into a "barnyard adventure"! This activity is a great way to introduce your new theme. Write a message (see sample below) on chart paper or a dry erase board each morning. As you write, invite children to help you sound out words, spell words, and decide what to write. Create a "secret code," and write a "secret message" for children to decode each day. Write the alphabet, and write a number above each letter (e.g., A–1, Z–26), or put numbers below your posted alphabet. Beneath the morning message, draw a blank and a number for each letter of the secret message (What animal is pink?).

Dear Farm Friends in Room ___,
Today is Tuesday, March ___, 200___.
Come with me to visit the farm!
Can you read my code?

___ ___ ___ ___
23 8   1   20

___ ___ ___ ___ ___
1 14   9 13   1 12

___ ___   ___ ___ ___ ___?
9 19   16   9 14 11

1	2	3	4	5	6	7
A	B	C	D	E	F	G
8	9	10	11	12	13	14
H	I	J	K	L	M	N
15	16	17	18	19	20	21
O	P	Q	R	S	T	U
22	23	24	25	26		
V	W	X	Y	Z		

Invite children to write in the room number and date with a marker or dry erase marker. Have them circle letters, words, or punctuation with a marker, a dry erase marker, or Wikki Stix. Depending on the level of the children, leave complete words or word chunks deleted for them to fill in. Have volunteers write the missing letters in the coded message. Have children read aloud the completed message. Choose a child to be the "farmer of the day," and invite him or her to use a reading stick (see page 19) to track and reread the morning message.

Pocket Chart Stories

Ⓜ Ⓐ Ⓣ Ⓔ Ⓡ Ⓘ Ⓐ Ⓛ Ⓢ

✓ mini-book reproducibles
   (pages 20–23 and 24–27)
✓ sentence strips
✓ colored markers
✓ pocket chart
✓ sticky notes

Choose a mini-book, and write each sentence on a separate sentence strip. Highlight key words by writing them in a different color to help children easily recognize them. Place the sentence strips in a pocket chart. Make copies of the mini-book pictures, color them, and place each picture next to the matching sentence. Have the class read aloud the story while you track and stress high-frequency words. Invite the class to revisit the story. Select a word, letter, or part of a word, and cover it with a sticky note. Invite children to use reading strategies to identify the selected word. Remind them to look at the beginning sound and to decide if their answer makes sense in the sentence.

Sentence Puzzle

Ⓜ Ⓐ Ⓣ Ⓔ Ⓡ Ⓘ Ⓐ Ⓛ Ⓢ

✓ sentence strips
✓ pocket chart

Choose a sentence strip from the pocket chart story (see above), and cut it apart to create word cards. Pass out the cards, and have children read aloud their word. Invite children with word cards to stand up and arrange their words so they form a sentence. Have them put the cards back in the pocket chart in the correct order.

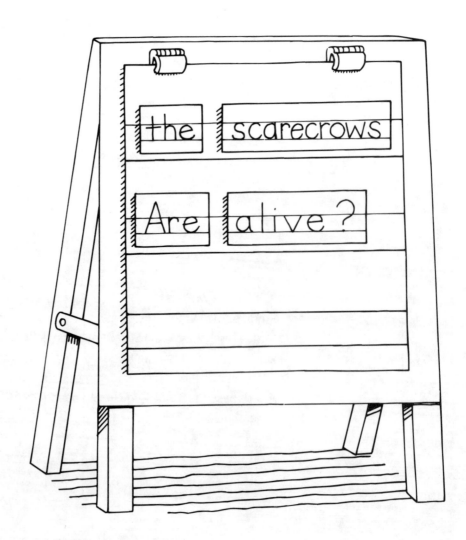

Guided Reading

Assembling the Mini-Books and Reading Sticks

MATERIALS

✓ mini-book reproducibles (pages 20–23 and 24–27)
✓ construction paper
✓ close-up photo of each child's face
✓ craft sticks
✓ stickers or small objects (e.g., bee, pig, tractor, scarecrow)
✓ envelopes

Make single-sided copies of the reproducibles for each mini-book. Fold each page in half so the blank side of the paper does not show, and staple the pages inside a construction paper cover so that the creased sides face out. Glue a photo of each child's face on the farmer on the last page of each book, or have children draw their face.

Reading sticks help children with one-to-one correspondence and left-to-right directionality and are fun to use. To make a reading stick, glue to the end of a craft stick a sticker or small object that relates to the theme of the mini-book. For example, use a bee for *Buzz, Buzz* and a pig, tractor, or scarecrow for *Are They Alive?* Seal envelopes, and cut them in half. Glue each envelope to the front inside cover of a mini-book to make a "pocket." Place a reading stick in the pocket.

Sight Word Practice

MATERIALS

✓ assembled mini-books (see above)
✓ assembled reading sticks (see above)
✓ art supplies

After children review the mini-book text in a shared reading lesson (see page 18), have them write the missing sight words in the blanks to complete their mini-book. In *Buzz, Buzz*, the sight word is *said*. Have children write their name as the farmer's name on page 8 in addition to the sight word. In *Are They Alive?*, the sight word is *are*. Invite children to decorate their covers and color the illustrations in their books. Have children use reading sticks to help them track words as they read the stories in guided reading groups.

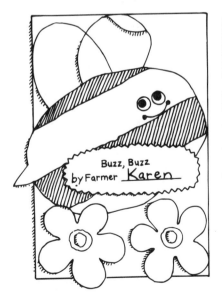

Buzz, Buzz
by Farmer Karen

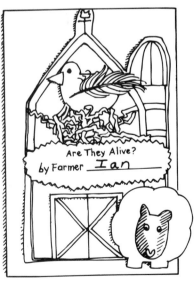

Are They Alive?
by Farmer Ian

Buzz, Buzz

by
Farmer

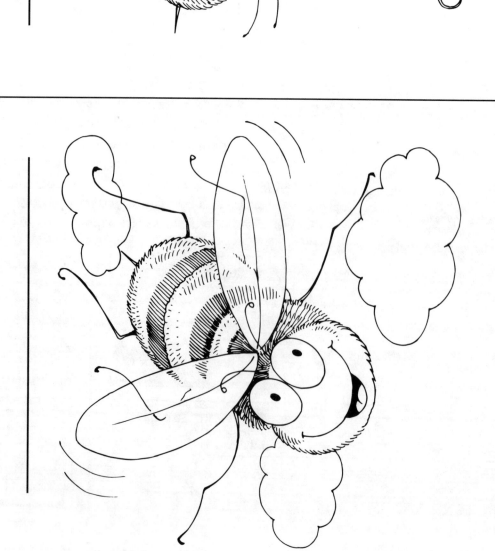

Dedicated to

2

"Buzz, buzz,"
_____ the bee.

"Moo, moo," _____
the cow.

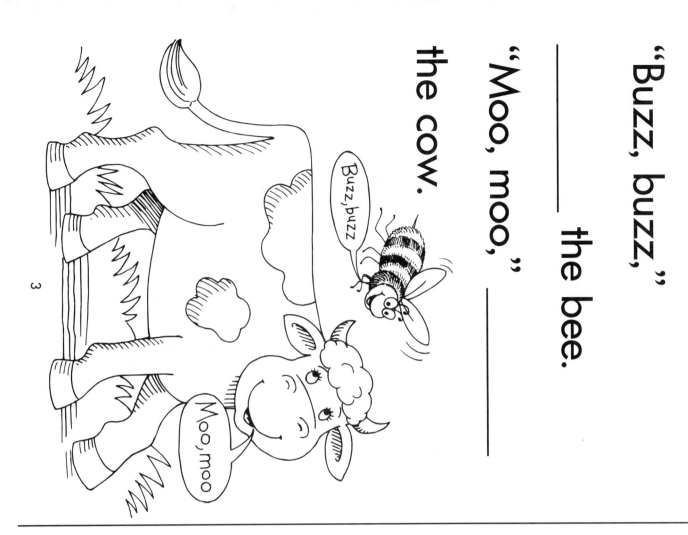

3

"Buzz, buzz,"
_____ the bee.

"Neigh, neigh," _____
the horse.

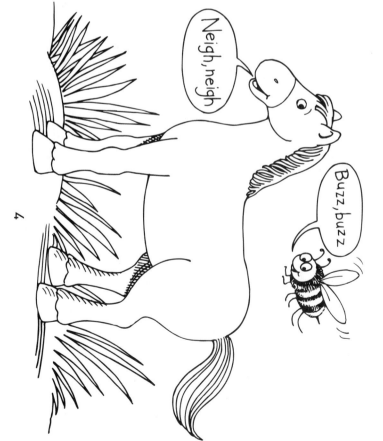

4

Down on the Farm © 2003 Creative Teaching Press

"Buzz, buzz,"
_____ the bee.

"Oink, oink,"
the pig. _____

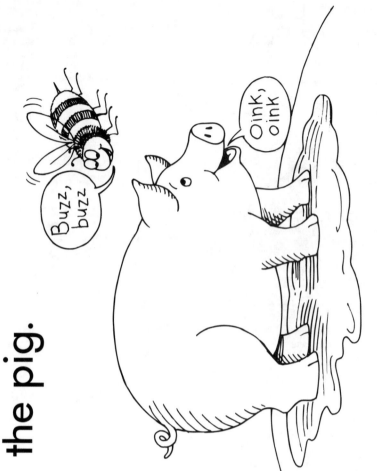

6

"Buzz, buzz,"
_____ the bee.

"Quack, quack,"
the duck. _____

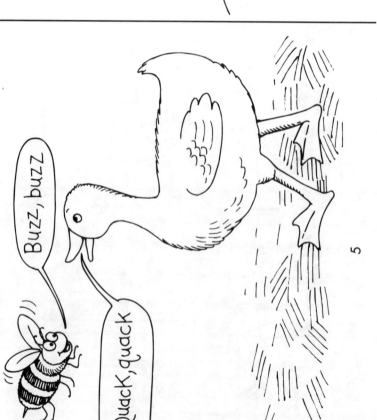

5

"Buzz, buzz," _____ the bee.

"Baa, baa," _____ the sheep.

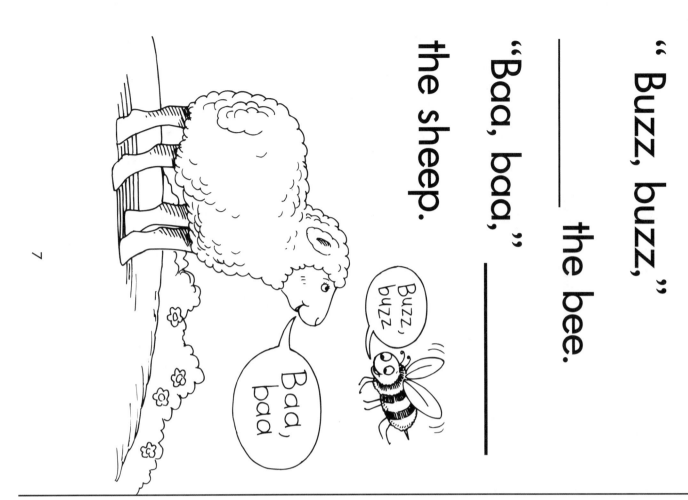

7

"Buzz, buzz," _____ the bee.

"Ouch!" _____ Farmer _____.

"You stung me!"

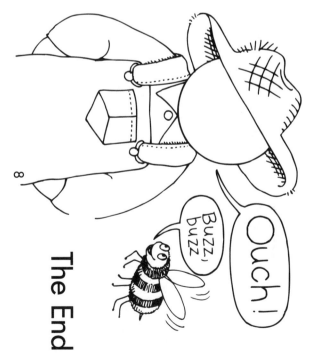

The End

8

Are They Alive?

by
Farmer

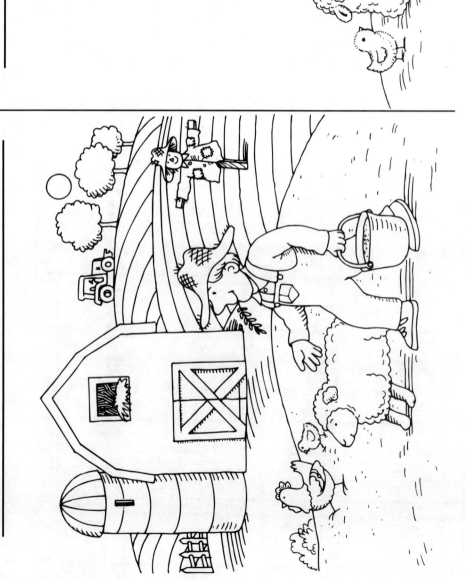

Dedicated to

2

_____ the barns alive?

No, they _____ not!

3

_____ the chickens alive?

Yes, they _____!

4

Down on the Farm © 2003 Creative Teaching Press

———— the sheep alive?

Yes, they ————!

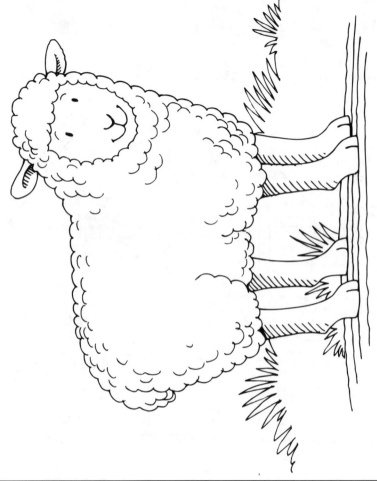

6

———— the scarecrows alive?

No, they ———— not!

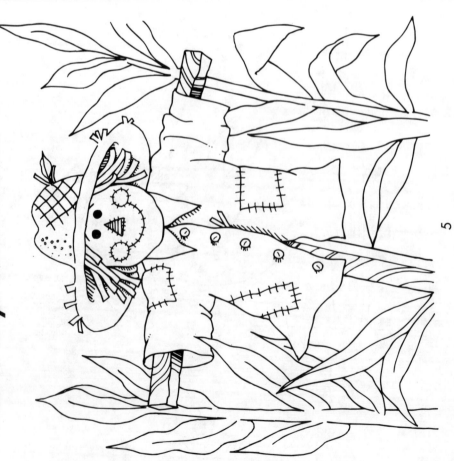

5

_____ the tractors _____ alive?

No, they _____ not!

7

_____ we alive?

Yes, we _____!

The End

8

Independent Reading

Professional Piggy Pack

MATERIALS

✓ *Career Day* by Anne Rockwell and *Jobs People Do* by Christopher Maynard

✓ Piggy Family Letter (page 29)

✓ Professional Piggy reproducible (page 30)

✓ construction paper

✓ pig stuffed animal

✓ small blanket

✓ backpack

Copy the Piggy Family Letter, which introduces the Professional Piggy Pack and explains how children will use its contents. Staple a class set of copies of the Professional Piggy reproducible inside a construction paper cover to make a Piggy Journal. Glue the letter to the cover. Place the journal, the books, a stuffed pig, and a blanket in a backpack. Send home the backpack with a different child each night. On the following day, have the child share his or her page of the journal with the class.

Down on the Silly Farm

MATERIALS

✓ Down on the Silly Farm reproducible (page 31)

✓ Farm Animals reproducible (page 14)

✓ Farmer reproducible (page 33)

✓ sentence strips

✓ color transparency of farmyard

✓ overhead projector

Invite your class to perform a dramatic play. Read aloud the play on the Down on the Silly Farm reproducible to introduce children to the characters and their lines. Assign every child a part. Make copies of the Farmer reproducible and enlarged copies of the Farm Animals reproducible. Give each child the corresponding cutout to color. (Have farmers draw a face on their cutout.) Invite children to glue their character cutout to a sentence strip to make a headband. Project the transparency onto a blank wall as the backdrop for the dramatic play. Have children practice their lines until they know them and are ready to perform in front of an audience.

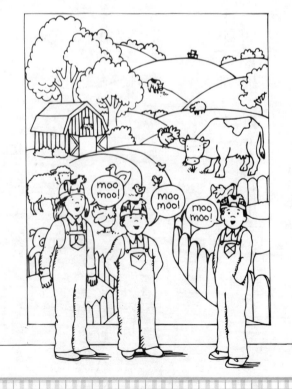

Piggy Family Letter

Dear Family,

Today your child has been a super citizen and is bringing home the Professional Piggy Pack! Have your child read the enclosed books about careers to you or with you. Have your child choose a profession for Piggy and complete a page in the Piggy Journal. Your child should write his or her name and the profession in the sentence frame (e.g., Ozzie's piggy is a doctor.) and decorate the pig so it looks as if it works in the chosen profession. Be creative! Invite your child to use fabric, wrapping paper, ribbon, or any other materials to decorate the pig on the journal page.

Please return all of the items in the backpack for another super citizen to take home tomorrow.

Have fun!

Sincerely,

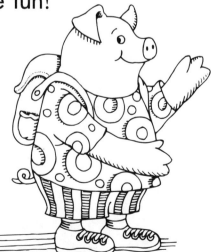

Professional Piggy

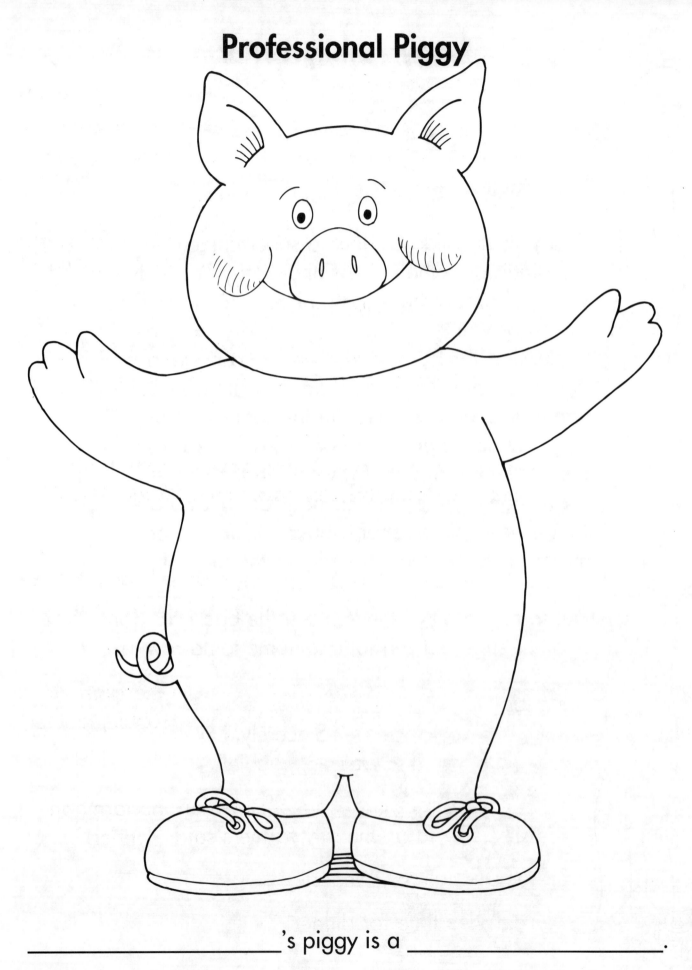

_____ 's piggy is a _____.

Down on the Silly Farm

(can be read to the tune of "Down by the Bay")

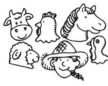 Cows, Horses, Sheep, Chickens, Turkeys, Farmers: Down on the farm, on the silly, silly farm, the silly pigs said, "Poink, poink!"

 Pigs: Oh, no! It's "Oink, oink!"

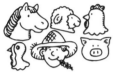 Horses, Sheep, Chickens, Turkeys, Farmers, Pigs: Down on the farm, on the silly, silly farm, the silly cows said, "Koo, koo!"

 Cows: Oh, no! It's "Moo, moo!"

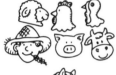 Sheep, Chickens, Turkeys, Farmers, Pigs, Cows: Down on the farm, on the silly, silly farm, the silly horses said, "Heigh, heigh!"

 Horses: Oh, no! It's "Neigh, neigh!"

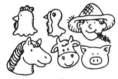 Chickens, Turkeys, Farmers, Pigs, Cows, Horses: Down on the farm, on the silly, silly farm, the silly sheep said, "Shaa, shaa!"

 Sheep: Oh, no! It's "Baa, baa!"

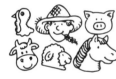 Turkeys, Farmers, Pigs, Cows, Horses, Sheep: Down on the farm, on the silly, silly farm, the silly chickens said, "Chuck, chuck!"

 Chickens: Oh, no! It's "Cluck, cluck!"

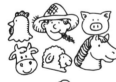 Farmers, Pigs, Cows, Horses, Sheep, Chickens: Down on the farm, on the silly, silly farm, the silly turkeys said, "Tobble, tobble!"

 Turkeys: Oh, no! It's "Gobble, gobble!"

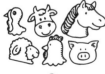 Pigs, Cows, Horses, Sheep, Chickens, Turkeys: Down on the farm, on the silly, silly farm, the silly farmers said, "Finner!"

 Farmers: Oh, no! It's "Dinner!"

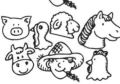 All: Yeah! It's time for dinner!

Shared Writing

Horsing Around with Words

✓ butcher paper
✓ yarn
✓ construction paper
✓ colored markers

Create a farm word bank with your class. Draw a large horse on butcher paper, and glue on yarn for its mane. Have children help you spell names of farm animals and key words such as *barn*, *haystack*, and *pond*. Write each word in bold dark colors on a piece of construction paper, and cut it out in its lettered shape. (Write vowels in a different color to help children identify them.) Glue these words to your horse, and display it on a classroom wall for whole-class reference. Reread the word bank words for a daily shared reading experience. Remind children to refer to these words during writing activities.

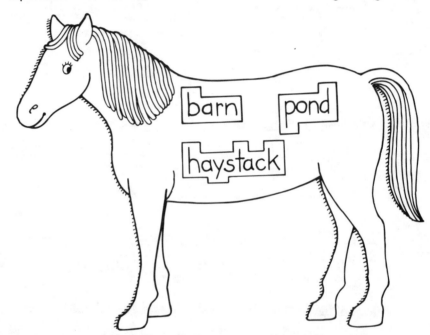

On the Farm

✓ Farmer reproducible (page 33)
✓ large sheets of lined paper
✓ construction paper
✓ straw hat
✓ close-up photo of each child's face
✓ art supplies

Staple a class set of lined paper between a construction paper cover to make a class Big Book. Write *On the Farm* on the cover. (Optional: Glue the Barn reproducible from page 9 on the book cover.) Each day, choose a different child to wear a straw hat and pretend to be a farmer. Ask children the same questions each day to complete the following sentence frames: *Farmer _____ feeds the _____. Farmer _____ plants _____. Farmer _____ likes to _____.* Write each child's responses on a separate page in the book. Ask children to help you sound out the words to spell them. Give each child a Farmer reproducible. Invite children to color their farmer, cut it out, glue their photo on it, and glue it next to their responses in the class book. Each day, begin the activity by rereading the previous days' pages for shared reading.

Farmer

Interactive Writing

Piggy Pete

MATERIALS

✓ nonfiction books about pigs
✓ sentence strips
✓ butcher paper
✓ newspaper
✓ art supplies

Read aloud books about pigs. Use interactive writing to have children take turns writing facts about pigs on sentence strips. Have volunteers take turns writing a letter, word chunk, whole word, or punctuation mark. For a fun way to display the pig facts, draw and cut out two large butcher paper pigs. Sponge-paint the pigs pink, glue them together, and stuff the pig with newspaper. Glue the sentence strips to the pig, and display it. Have children read the facts in small groups for ongoing shared reading.

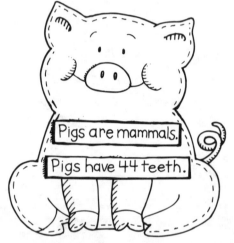

Pigs are mammals.

Pigs have 44 teeth.

Farm Fun Number Poem

MATERIALS

✓ chart paper
✓ sentence strips
✓ butcher paper

Have children brainstorm names of farm animals, and record them on chart paper. Then, have children brainstorm words that rhyme with the numbers 1–10. Use interactive writing to have children write a poem (see sample poem below) on separate sentence strips. Have them use a word from each list to write each line. Invite volunteers to share in the writing process for each line. Reread the poem for shared reading. Then, mount the sentence strips on large sheets of butcher paper to make a Big Book, and have children illustrate each page.

1, 1 Farm fun

2, 2 Horses for you

3, 3 Bees in a tree

4, 4 Pigs want more

5, 5 Ducks can dive

6, 6 Chicks in sticks

7, 7 Sheep look at heaven

8, 8 Cows by the gate

9, 9 It's time to dine

10, 10 It's night again

Guided Writing

On the Silly Farm

Copy the On the Silly Farm reproducible for every two children, and cut apart the sentence frames. Copy a class set of the Barn reproducible on red construction paper, and copy a class set of the Farmer reproducible. Read aloud *Cock-A-Doodle-Moo!* Invite children to brainstorm a list of farm animals. Have children help you sound them out and spell them as you record them on chart paper. (You can draw a picture next to each animal name as a reading cue.) Give each child a sentence frame, a copy of each reproducible, and a butcher paper square. Have children write their name and the name of a farm animal in the first two blanks of the sentence frame. Have them use the beginning sound of their animal's name to replace the beginning sounds of *Cock-a-doodle-doo!* For example, if a child chose a sheep, he or she would write **Sh**ock-a-**sh**oodle-**sh**oo! Have children color and cut out their Barn reproducible. Ask children to draw a face on the Farmer reproducible and then color it and cut it out. Ask them to paint the animal they wrote about and cut it out. Have children glue their sentence frame, barn, farmer, and animal on their square. Bind the squares together to make a Big Book for children to read independently, or display the squares on a bulletin board.

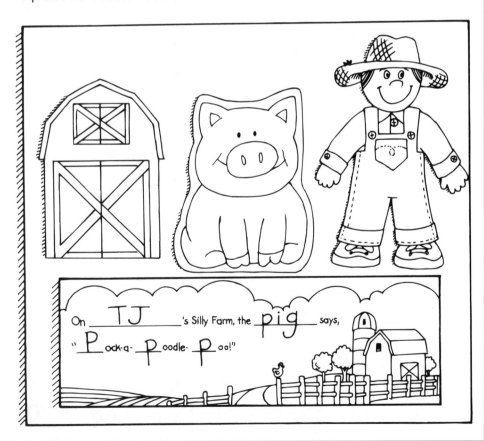

On ___TJ___'s Silly Farm, the ___pig___ says, "___P___ock-a-___P___oodle-___P___oo!"

On the Silly Farm

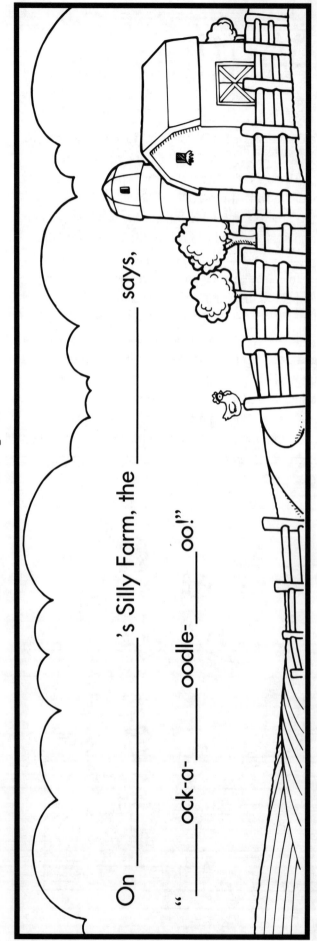

On _____'s Silly Farm, the _____ says,

"_____ock-a-_____oodle-_____oo!"

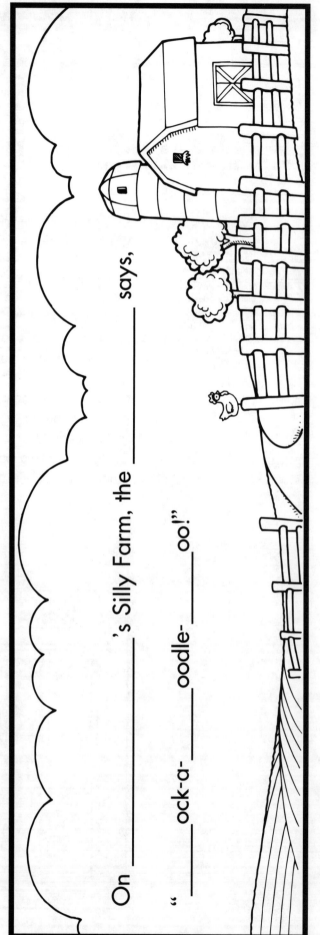

On _____'s Silly Farm, the _____ says,

"_____ock-a-_____oodle-_____oo!"

Wishy-Washy Bathtub

MATERIALS

✓ *Mrs. Wishy-Washy* by Joy Cowley
✓ Bathtub reproducible (page 38)
✓ Farmer reproducible (page 33)
✓ construction paper
✓ art supplies

Read aloud *Mrs. Wishy-Washy*. Invite children to paint the head of a farm animal on white construction paper, and cut it out. Give each child a Bathtub reproducible, and have children cut out the bathtub. Have children write the name of their animal in the first blank of the sentence frame. Then, have them write the first letter of the animal's name in the following blanks (e.g., *In went the horse. Hishy-hashy. Hishy-hashy*). Give each child a Farmer reproducible. Have children cut out the farmer, trace it on white construction paper, and decorate it to look like themselves. Then, have children cut out their farmer and glue it to the back of the bathtub (at one end) so only the top of the body is showing above the bubbles. Tell children to glue the farm animal head at the other end so it appears that they are taking a bath with the animal. Ask children to glue their bathtub on a sheet of construction paper. Invite the class to read aloud with you each child's sentence frame. Before reading each one, have children name the animal in the picture, the letter it starts with, and the sound that letter makes. Remind children to replace the *w* in *wishy-washy* with the first letter of the animal's name as they read the sentence frame. Display children's work around the classroom.

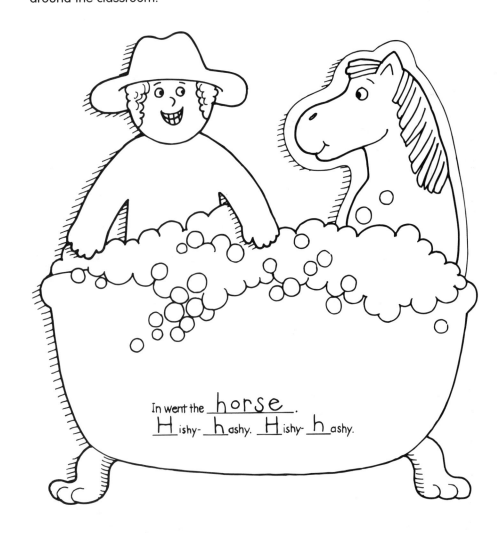

In went the _horse_.
_H_ishy- _h_ashy. _H_ishy- _h_ashy.

Bathtub

In went the _____ .

_____ ishy-_____ ashy.

_____ ishy-_____ ashy.

Independent Writing

Nibbling Rabbit Mural

(M)(A)(T)(E)(R)(I)(A)(L)(S)

✓ *The Tale of Peter Rabbit* by Beatrix Potter
✓ sentence strips
✓ butcher paper
✓ art supplies

Read aloud *The Tale of Peter Rabbit.* Have each child brainstorm one to three foods that begin with the same sound as their first name. Ask children to choose one of the foods and write a sentence about a rabbit eating that food (e.g., *Luca's rabbit nibbles lettuce*) on a sentence strip. Invite children to paint a watercolor picture of a rabbit in a garden eating the food they wrote about. Make a mural of a garden on butcher paper, and title it *Down in the Garden by the Little Rabbits in Room ___.* Attach each child's painting and sentence strip to the mural, and display it. Encourage children to independently read each other's sentences.

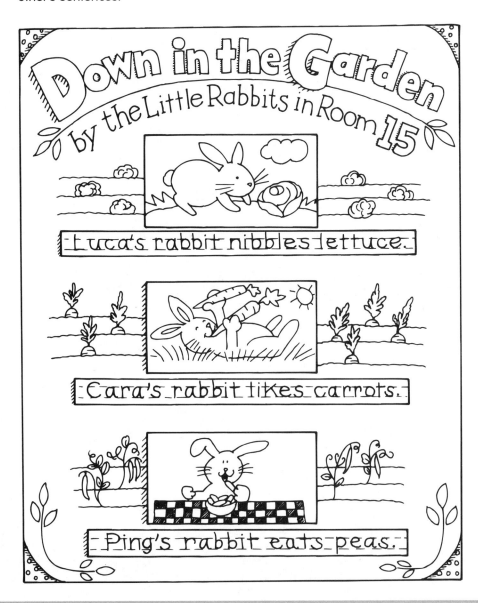

Down in the Garden by the Little Rabbits in Room 15

Luca's rabbit nibbles lettuce.

Cara's rabbit likes carrots.

Ping's rabbit eats peas.

Piggy Tales

MATERIALS

- ✓ *Pigs in the Mud in the Middle of the Rud* by Lynn Plourde
- ✓ Pig reproducible (page 41)
- ✓ Piggy Tales reproducible (page 42)
- ✓ tagboard
- ✓ wiggly eyes
- ✓ pipe cleaners
- ✓ sponges cut in 1" (2.5 cm) squares
- ✓ brown butcher paper
- ✓ art supplies

Make several copies of the Pig reproducible on tagboard, and cut them out to make patterns for a pig head and a pig body. Read aloud *Pigs in the Mud in the Middle of the Rud.* Invite children to discuss facts about pigs. Have children write facts about pigs (e.g., *Pigs like corn, Pigs roll in the mud*) on the Piggy Tales reproducible. Encourage children to write on additional writing templates (if necessary), and then staple together each child's papers. Have children trace the pig head and cut it out. Then, have children fold a piece of 9" x 12" (23 cm x 30.5 cm) tagboard in half and trace the pig body so the top of the body is on the fold. Invite children to cut out the body without unfolding the tagboard. (They may need adult help.) Tell them not to cut on the fold line. Have children paint their pig, add wiggly eyes and a pipe cleaner tail, and glue their writing inside of the pig body. Then, have children glue a sponge to the back of their pig head and glue the sponge to the pig body. Cut out a "mud puddle" from brown butcher paper, and display the pigs on it.

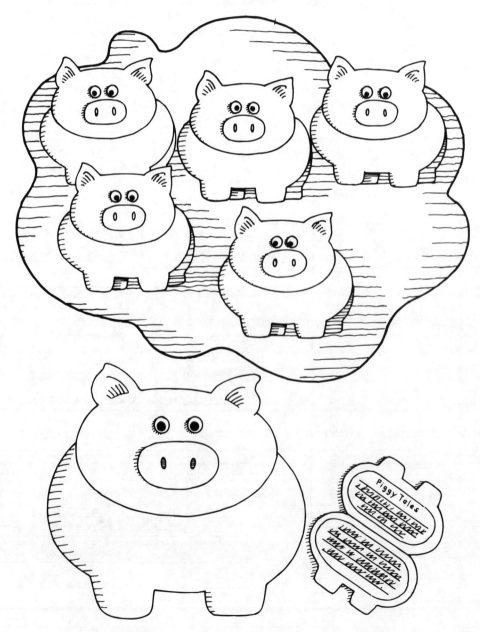

Pig

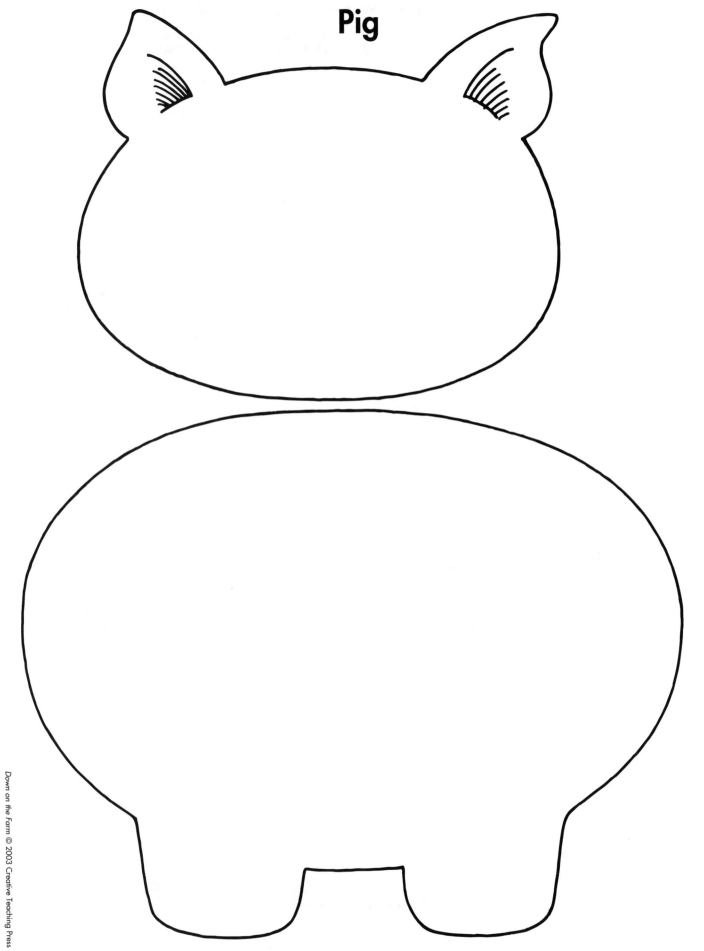

Piggy Tales

_____

_____

_____

_____

_____

_____

_____

_____

_____

_____

_____

_____

_____

_____

_____

Math

Mr. Horse's Tasty Treats

MATERIALS

✓ butcher paper
✓ picture of a horse (optional)
✓ fresh vegetables (broccoli, carrots, cauliflower, tomatoes)
✓ pictures of vegetables (optional)
✓ sentence strips
✓ art supplies

Draw a large cartoon horse on butcher paper, and cut it out. Or, glue a picture of a horse to the top of a large butcher paper square. Gather fresh vegetables for children to taste, and draw them at the bottom of the horse (or glue pictures of them on the horse). Invite children to taste the vegetables and choose which one is their favorite. Have children draw this vegetable, cut it out, and glue it on the horse above the matching picture to create a bar graph. Use interactive writing to have children write the rhyme *Old Mr. Horse, what do you like with hay: broccoli, carrots, cauliflower, or tomatoes on this lovely day?* Display the graph and the rhyme on a wall, and invite children to analyze the data. Use interactive writing to record on separate sentence strips the information children share about the graph, and display them near the horse. For example, children may say *Cauliflower is 1 person's favorite vegetable, More people like carrots than tomatoes,* or *The same number of people like broccoli and carrots.*

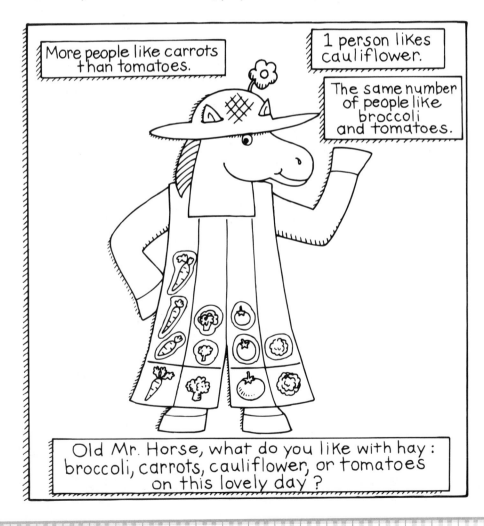

More people like carrots than tomatoes.

1 person likes cauliflower.

The same number of people like broccoli and tomatoes.

Old Mr. Horse, what do you like with hay : broccoli, carrots, cauliflower, or tomatoes on this lovely day ?

Watermelon Seed Number Book

MATERIALS

✓ Watermelon reproducible (page 45)
✓ construction paper
✓ black beans
✓ small paper plates
✓ art supplies

Make enough copies of the Watermelon reproducible for each child to practice counting. For example, if children are practicing counting from 0–5, make three copies for each child for a total of six watermelons. Staple a set of pages inside a construction paper cover to make a number book for each child. Invite children to write each number in large bold print above or below each watermelon on a separate page. Then, have them glue the corresponding number of black beans (watermelon seeds) on each watermelon. Encourage children to practice counting by rereading their book. Have children write on the cover _____'s *Watermelon Seed Counting Book*. Then, have them cut a small paper plate in half, paint it green and red, and glue black beans on it so it looks like a watermelon. Ask them to glue their plate on their book cover. To extend the activity to include addition or subtraction, give children two colors of beans. Invite them to glue two colors of "seeds" on their watermelon, write an addition equation above or below each watermelon, and count how many seeds they have in all. For subtraction, have children put a chosen number of seeds on the watermelon, remove some, and then put them next to the watermelon. Tell children to glue the seeds on their paper, write a subtraction equation, and solve it.

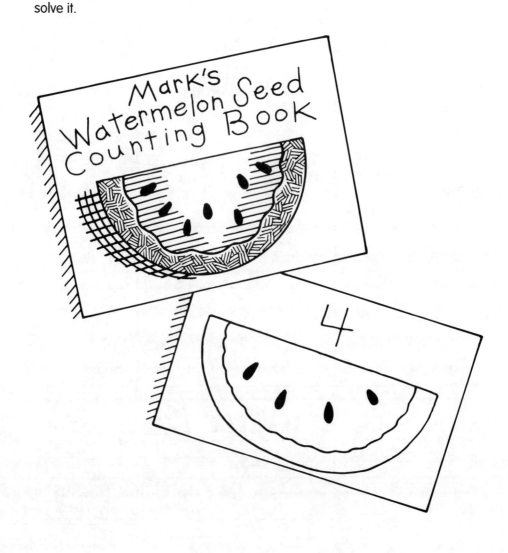

Watermelon

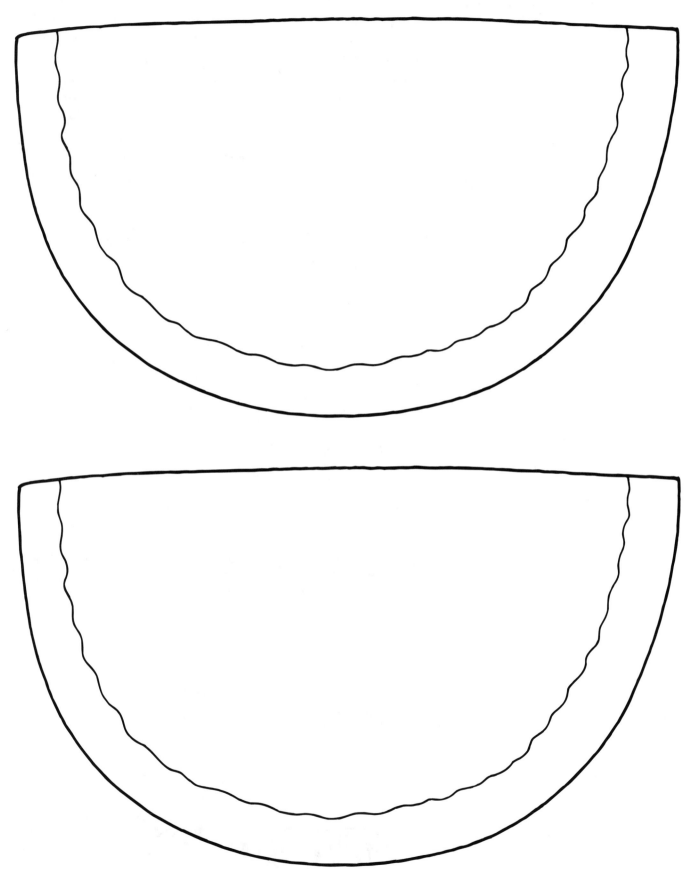

Scarecrow Glyph

(M A T E R I A L S)

✓ Scarecrow Glyph Key
  reproducible (page 47)
✓ construction paper
✓ buttons
✓ plastic flowers
✓ fabric squares
✓ art supplies

Copy the Scarecrow Glyph Key reproducible, mount it on construction paper, and display it. Give each child assorted colors of construction paper. Have children cut construction paper to make a scarecrow head, body, overalls, and a hat, and have them glue the pieces together (see sample below). Have children refer to the glyph key to add details to their scarecrow. If the child is a girl, have her glue a flower on her scarecrow's hat. Have children glue on their scarecrow button eyes that are the same color as their own eyes. Ask children to add a triangle nose to represent whether they prefer carrots or peas. Then, have them glue on the overalls the same number of patches (fabric squares) as how old they are (e.g., five years old = five patches). Display the scarecrows in the classroom, and have children use the key to analyze the data on each scarecrow. For example, a child might say *Paolo is a boy because he doesn't have a flower on his scarecrow's hat. His eyes are green because the scarecrow has green button eyes. His scarecrow has an orange nose so he must like to eat carrots more than peas. Paolo is six years old because his scarecrow has six patches on its overalls.*

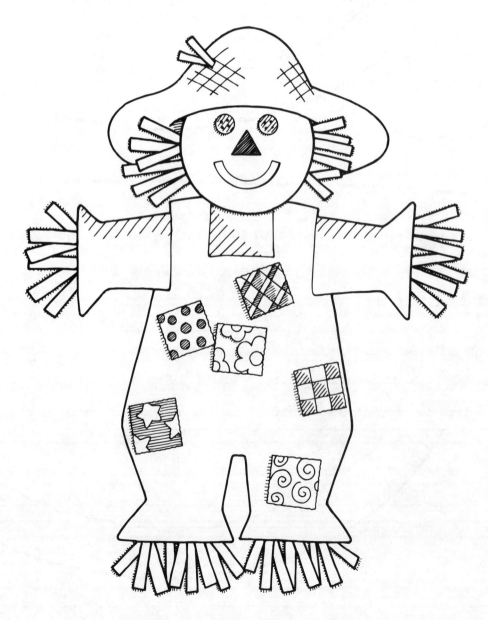

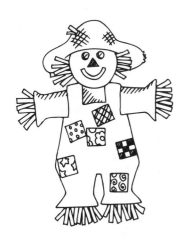

Scarecrow Glyph Key

1 <u>Are you a boy or a girl</u>?
Boys: Do not glue a flower on the hat.
Girls: Glue a flower on the hat.

2 <u>What color are your eyes</u>?
Give the scarecrow button eyes the same color as your eyes.

3 <u>Do you like to eat carrots or peas better</u>?
Make an orange triangle nose if you like to eat carrots.

Make a green triangle nose if you like to eat peas.

4 <u>How old are you</u>?
Glue on to the overalls the same number of patches as how old you are.

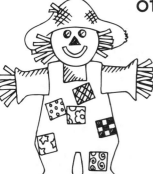

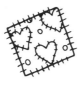
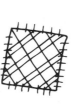

Addition Nests

Ⓜ Ⓐ Ⓣ Ⓔ Ⓡ Ⓘ Ⓐ Ⓛ Ⓢ

✓ Birds reproducible (page 49)
✓ small plastic eggs
✓ brown paper bags
✓ plastic grass
✓ craft sticks
✓ art supplies

Give each child a Birds reproducible and a handful of plastic eggs. Invite children to color and cut out the birds. Have children choose one or two birds and a number of eggs to add together. Tell them to write these two numbers in the frame on their reproducible and then write an addition equation. Invite children to roll down the top of a paper bag to make a "bird's nest" and sponge-paint it. Have them glue their frame on the side of the bag. Invite children to fill their bag with plastic grass. Then, have children glue their bird(s) on craft sticks and put them in the nest and put their egg(s) inside the nest. Encourage children to show their nest to the class and explain their equation. To extend the activity, mount the equation frames on construction paper, and laminate the papers. Have children use the birds and eggs to create several different addition combinations. Have them use an overhead marker to write numbers in the blanks.

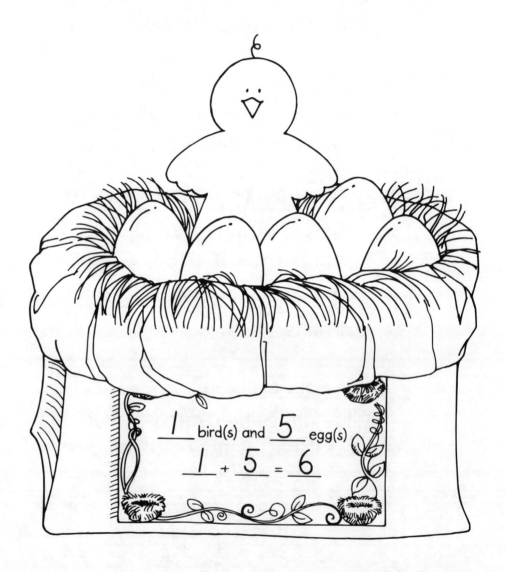

___1___ bird(s) and ___5___ egg(s)

$$1 + 5 = 6$$

Birds

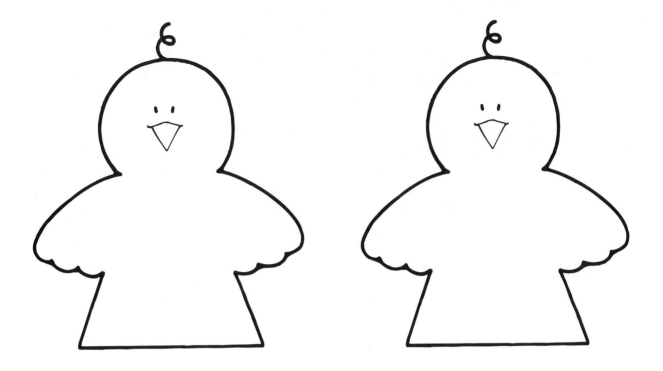

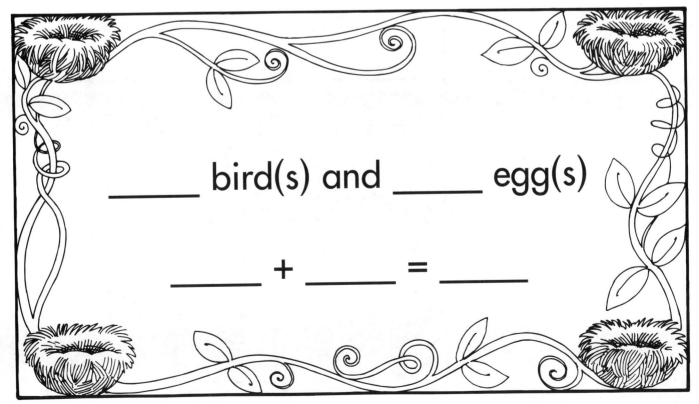

_____ bird(s) and _____ egg(s)

_____ + _____ = _____

Ants on a Picnic

Copy a class set of the Ants reproducible on red construction paper. Choose a number that children will use as the sum in addition problems. Make enough copies of the Picnic reproducible for each child to make a book with one page for each addition problem. For example, if you choose the number 5, give children six pages so they can write and illustrate the equations $0 + 5 = 5$, $1 + 4 = 5$, $2 + 3 = 5$, $3 + 2 = 5$, $4 + 1 = 5$, and $5 + 0 = 5$. Assemble the books by stapling a set of Picnic reproducibles inside a green construction paper cover. Give each child an assembled book and enough copies of the Ants reproducible to complete a book. Have children cut apart the ants. On each page, have children glue a set of ants on the basket and a set of ants on the plate to equal the chosen number and then write the addition equation. Invite children to decorate their cover and write ____ ants on a picnic are not so great! ____ tiny ants are on my plate!

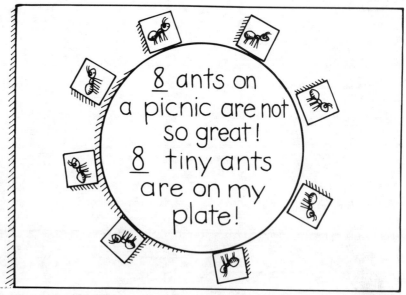

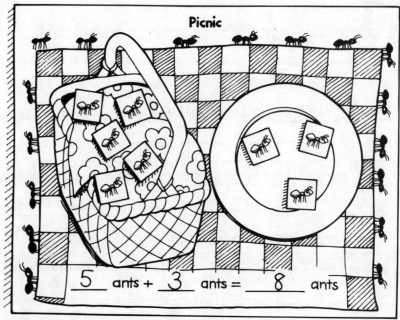

Ants

Picnic

_____ ants + _____ ants = _____ ants

Science

Seasons on the Farm

Cut two large white butcher paper circles for each child. Read aloud *The Seasons of Arnold's Apple Tree*. Discuss the seasons and different activities that take place on the farm during each season. Invite children to paint the earth on one of their circles. Cut a large *X* in the middle of each child's "earth" to create four flaps, and glue the outer edges of the earth to the second circle. Have children fold back each flap and write *fall, winter, spring*, and *summer* on the underside. Invite children to write a sentence about something related to the farm in each season on the white paper below each flap (e.g., fall—apple harvest, winter—snow on the barn, spring—baby chicks, summer—corn stalks) and illustrate it. Invite children to share their illustrations and sentences with the class.

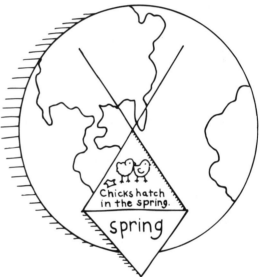

Plant a Sunflower Garden

Plant sunflower seeds in a large pot. Ask children to monitor the growth of the sunflowers. When children observe a change, record it on chart paper. Invite a volunteer to document the change by drawing the pot and plant on the chart paper and recording the date below the drawing. Invite children to plant their own sunflower. Poke a hole in the bottom of a plastic cup for each child. Have children add soil and five sunflower seeds to their cup. For a fun display, invite children to decorate their cup by gluing a construction paper wheelbarrow on the front of it. Have them draw and cut out a construction paper flower, glue the flower to a dowel, and stick it in the cup.

Social Studies

Who Will Help Me?

Make several copies of the Chef Hats reproducible on white construction paper, and cut them apart. Type in large print the following sentence frame: "*Who will help me _____?*" "*____ _____,*" *said _____*. Make eight copies of the sentence frames, and glue them to separate large sheets of construction paper to make pages for a Big Book. Read aloud *The Little Red Hen*, and discuss how no one wanted to help the hen. Ask children what the kinder thing to do would have been. Tell them it would have been nice if the animals had all said, "I will!" Display the Big Book pages, and use interactive writing to have children complete each sentence frame. For each page, have volunteers write in the first blank a different step for making cookies (e.g., *sift the flour, measure the sugar, mix the butter, crack the eggs, pour the milk, mix the chocolate chips, bake the cookies,* and *eat the cookies.*) Then, have the volunteers write *I will* and their name on the following lines. Have the children who helped write the information on the page glue their photo above the writing frame and glue a chef hat on their head in their photo. Have children illustrate their page with construction paper cutouts of their ingredients being put into a bowl. Staple together the completed pages. To extend the activity, have children make a batch of cookies. Or, invite children to write ways to help make other items (e.g., play dough, monster made from blocks).

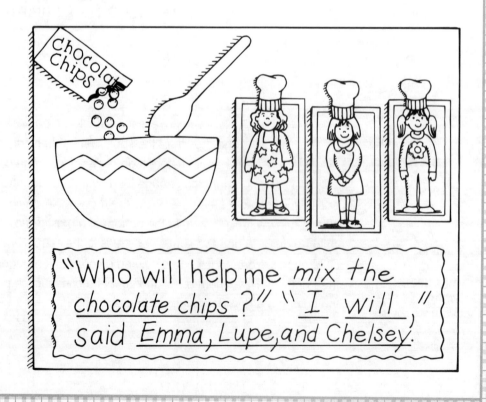

"Who will help me *mix the chocolate chips* ?" " *I will* ," said *Emma, Lupe, and Chelsey.*

Chef Hats

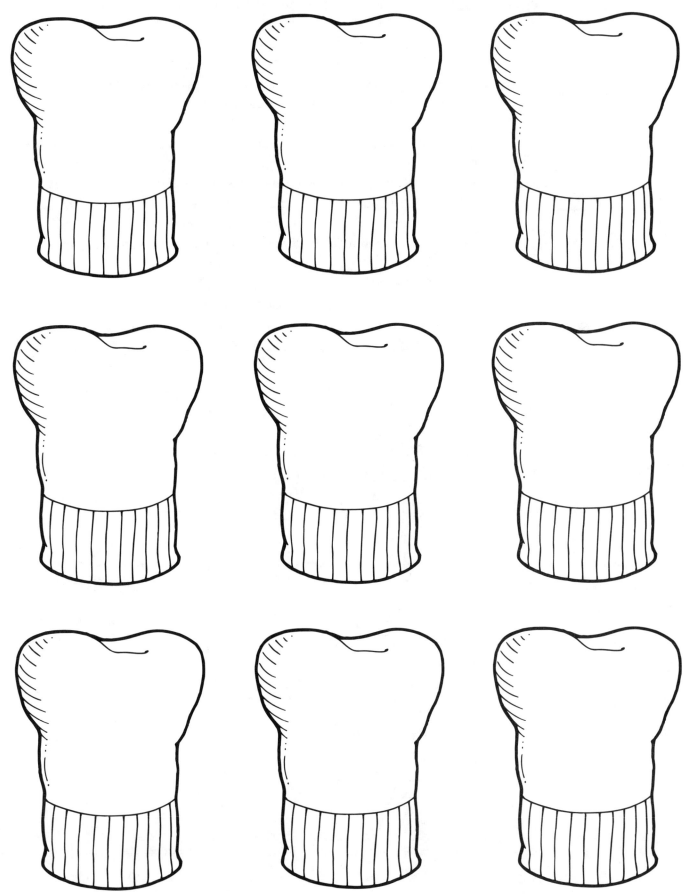

What Did You Grow?

(M)(A)(T)(E)(R)(I)(A)(L)(S)

✓ *Growing Vegetable Soup* by Lois Ehlert
✓ Vegetables reproducible (page 57)
✓ tagboard
✓ fresh vegetables (celery, corn, potato, beans)
✓ newspaper or paper towels
✓ large paper bags
✓ art supplies

Copy a class set of the Vegetables reproducible on tagboard. Read aloud *Growing Vegetable Soup.* Discuss what farmers grow and why produce is important. Show children fresh vegetables, and discuss the parts of the plant (stem, flower, root, seeds). Invite children to taste each food. Discuss how each vegetable grows (e.g., on a stalk, underground). Give each child a Vegetables reproducible. Have children cut out each vegetable, trace it on tagboard, and cut it out. Invite children to sponge-paint their vegetables (not over the sentence frame box). Have children complete each sentence frame. Tell children to glue together matching cutouts back-to-back and stuff them with newspaper or paper towels. Then, invite children to sponge-paint a large paper bag, fold down the bag to make it look like a basket, and staple a paper handle on it. Tell children to then put the stuffed food cutouts in their "basket." To extend the activity, have children write about why a farmer would grow products, why they are important, or how they are used. Invite children to complete the sentence frame *Farmer _____ grows _____, _____, and _____ because _____.* For example, a child might write *Farmer Shayna grows carrots, apples, and beans because they are healthy* or *Farmer Tim grows apples, strawberries, and pumpkins because they can be baked in pies and sold at the market.*

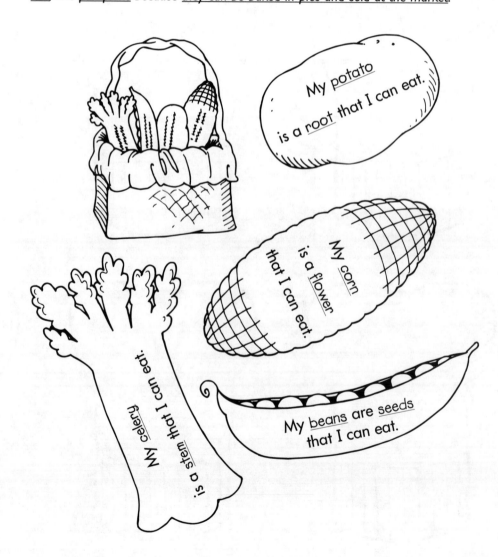

My potato is a <u>root</u> that I can eat.

My <u>corn</u> is a <u>flower</u> that I can eat.

My <u>beans</u> are seeds that I can eat.

My <u>celery</u> is a <u>stem</u> that I can eat.

Vegetables

My _____ that I can eat.

is a _____

My _____

is a _____

that I can eat.

My _____

is a _____ that I can eat.

My _____ are _____

that I can eat.

Culminating Event and Extra Fun

At the end of your unit, host an Evening on the Farm. Invite children and their families to visit the classroom so children can act as a guide to show off all the projects they completed during the unit and share the information they learned about the farm. Arrange your classroom so all the projects children completed are displayed. Prior to the event, have children practice leading a partner or small group around the classroom and explaining each project. This will help prepare children and make them feel confident when their family visits the classroom. Invite children to complete the following fun activities to provide decorations and props for the "big event."

Evening on the Farm Invitation

MATERIALS

✓ Apple Core reproducible (page 62)
✓ construction paper
✓ art supplies

Give each child an Apple Core reproducible copied on white construction paper. Invite children to write in the location, date, and time of the Evening on the Farm event. Have them cut out the apple core and color the stem brown and the leaf green. Have children cut out two circles (approximately 9" or 23 cm) to make two "apples" from red construction paper. Tell children to glue together the bottoms and sides of the apples to make an apple pocket. Then, have them slide their apple core inside of the apple. Tell children to bring home their apple with their apple core invitation inside it to give to their family.

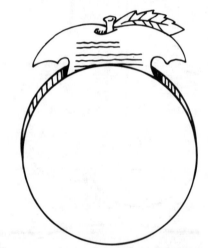

Farmer's Hat

MATERIALS

✓ large paper plates (hard or heavy-duty)
✓ paper bowls (hard or heavy-duty)
✓ hay or yellow construction paper strips
✓ art supplies

Cut a circle in the center of a large paper plate for each child. Glue a paper bowl upside down on the bottom of each plate to create a hat. Have children paint their hat and glue hay or yellow construction paper strips on it.

Cooking on the Farm

Gather for each child or small group the ingredients and materials listed on a recipe. Give each child a copy of the recipe. Have children follow the recipe and color each illustration. For extra fun, read *Piggy Pie!* by Margie Palatini to the class.

Papier-Mâché Rockin' Roosters

Cut out a class set of roosters from foam core board (see sample shape below). Glue them onto ½" (13 mm) thick dowels. Use a drill to make a hole in a block of wood for each child. Glue a dowel in the hole in each block. Cut newspaper or paper towels into small pieces. Invite children to dip the newspaper or paper towels in liquid starch and cover the foam board (usually two coatings are necessary) with the pieces to create a papier-mâché rooster. After the starch dries, have children paint their rooster, dowel, and wood base a solid color. Then, have them add polka dots and an orange construction paper beak to the rooster. Ask an adult to hot-glue feathers to each rooster to make a tail and red felt to make a wattle and a comb. Invite children to glue popcorn kernels to the wood base. (Option: Display roosters on top of bails of hay or boxes decorated to look like hay.)

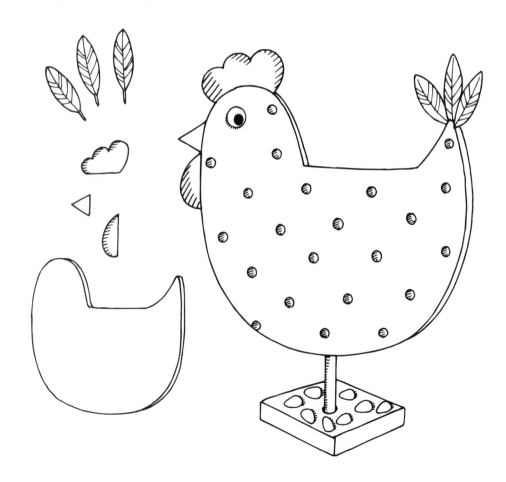

Hayride Hoedown Bulletin Board

MATERIALS

✓ butcher paper
✓ paper plates
✓ red bandanas or red fabric
✓ art supplies

Cover a bulletin board with blue butcher paper. Accordion-fold a piece of brown butcher paper with folds deep enough to hold paper vegetables, and staple it on the board so the folds look like rows in a field. Cut out a butcher paper tractor and two or three (depending on your class size) wagons, and staple them on the bulletin board as if they were driving across the dirt. Invite each child to paint a paper plate and add a face and hair. Cut red bandanas or fabric into triangles, and hang them like a scarf from each paper-plate "head." (Girls can add small pieces tied in bows in their hair.) Attach the heads to the wagons. Invite children to make paper vegetables and place them in the folds of the "dirt" to look like a field. Use interactive writing to have children write captions for what they would say as they rode along the field. Add the captions to the display. For example, children could write *This is fun!* or *What a bumpy ride!*

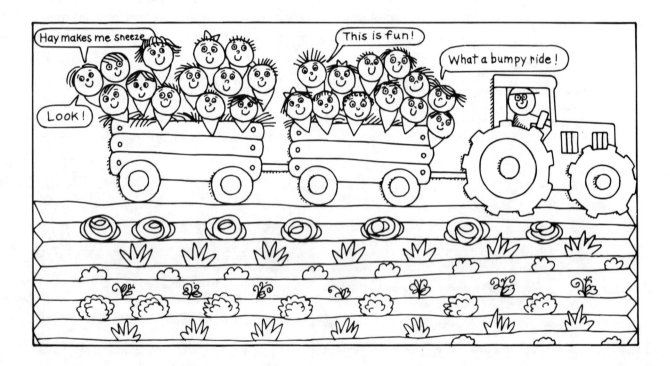

Midnight on the Farm Bulletin Board

MATERIALS

✓ black butcher paper
✓ paper plates
✓ construction paper
✓ art supplies

Cover a bulletin board with black butcher paper. Paint a tree, stars, and grass on the background. (Optional: Attach twinkle lights to the edge of the board.) Have children paint paper plates to make the heads of sleeping animals (i.e., yellow for ducks, pink for pigs, tan for cows). Have them cut out construction paper to create ears, closed eyes, beaks, and noses to add to the animal heads. Staple the completed animal heads on the bulletin board. Use interactive writing to have children write captions in speech bubbles to illustrate the noises sleeping animals might make, and staple them above the animals. For example, children could write *Zzz-oink!* above pigs, *Zzz-moo!* above cows, and *Zzz-quack!* above ducks.

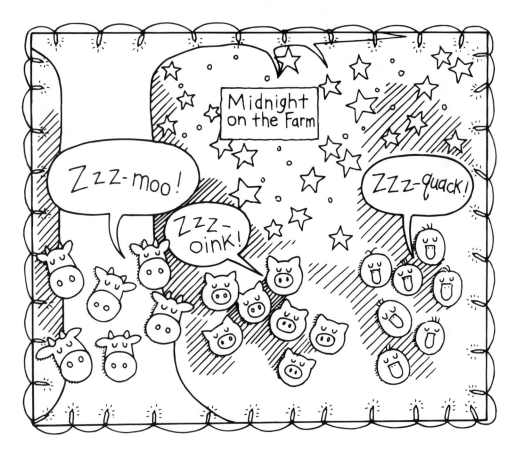

Apple Core

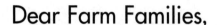

Dear Farm Families,

We have been busy turning our classroom into a fantastic farm! Your little farmer would love to have you come see all our projects.

Where: _____

When: _____

Time: _____

We can't wait to see you at our Evening on the Farm event!

Sincerely,

Farmer

_____

Sunflower Snacks Recipe

by Chef _____

> **Ingredients:** white frosting, round cracker,
> Hershey's Kiss®, candy corn,
> stick pretzel
>
> **Materials:** plastic knife, napkin

1 Spread white frosting on a round cracker.

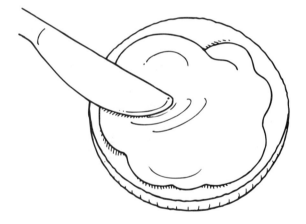

2 Place one chocolate kiss in the center.

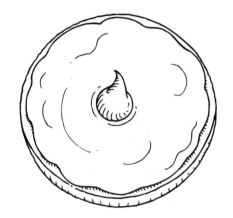

3 Place candy corn around the edges.

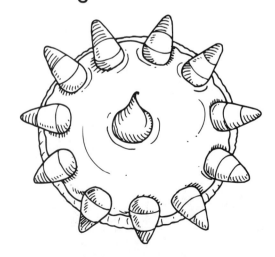

4 Add a pretzel stem.

Piggy Pie Recipe

by Chef _____

> <u>Ingredients</u>: graham cracker, chocolate pudding, chocolate chips, large marshmallow, pink sprinkles
>
> <u>Materials</u>: paper cupcake cup, plastic spoon

1 Smash a graham cracker into small pieces and put them in a cupcake cup.

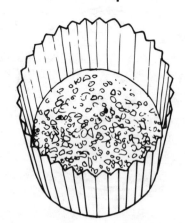

2 Add a scoop of chocolate pudding to make mud.

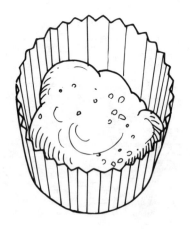

3 Put 4 chocolate chips (pig's feet) and a large marshmallow (pig) in the mud.

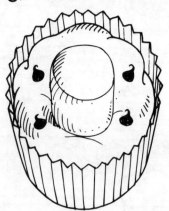

4 Add pink sprinkles to make pink piggy dust.

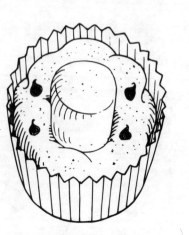